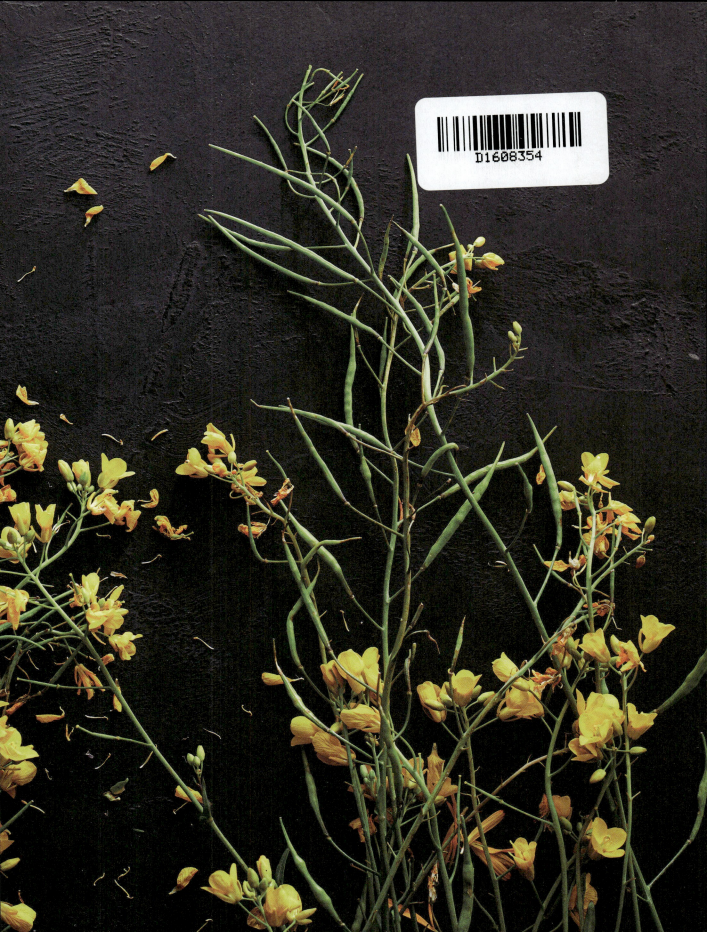

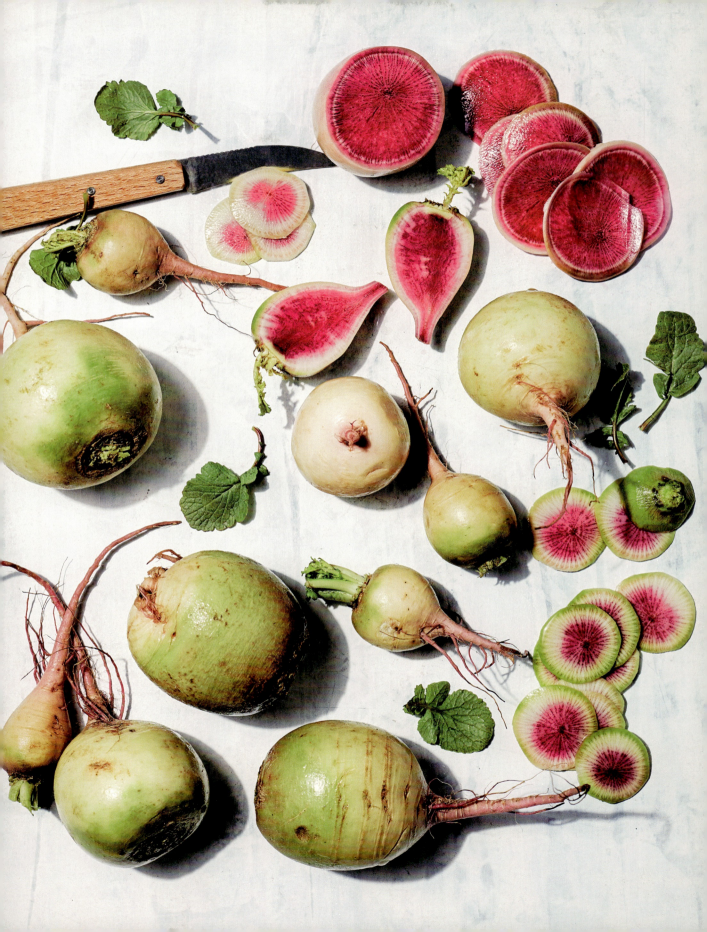

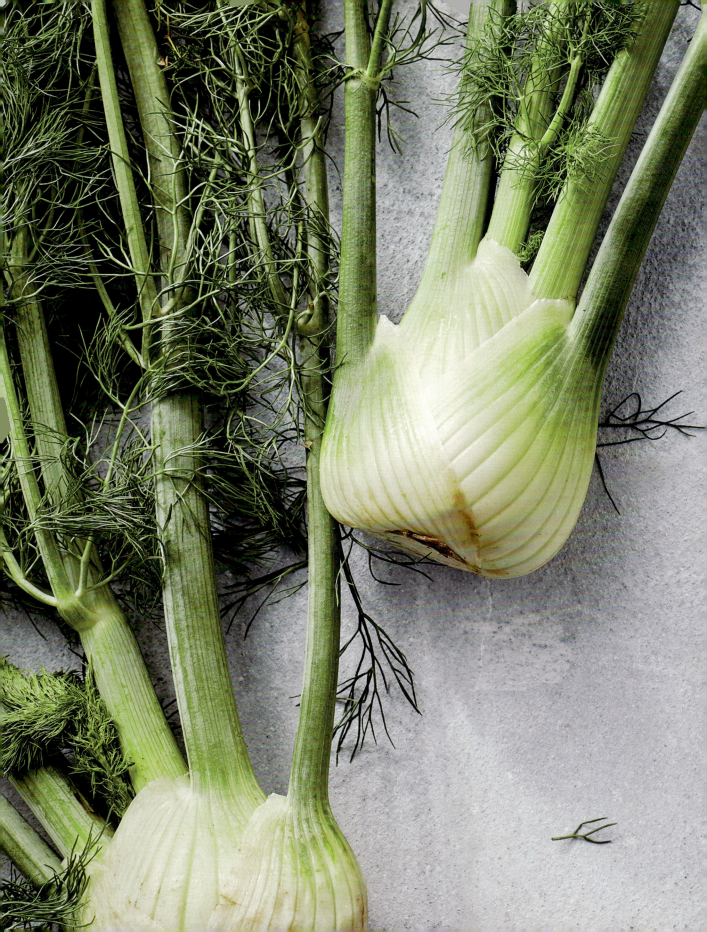

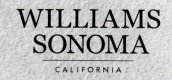

WILLIAMS
SONOMA

CALIFORNIA

EVERYDAY
healthy
COOKBOOK

DANA JACOBI

PHOTOGRAPHY BY
EVA KOLENKO

weldon**owen**

Contents

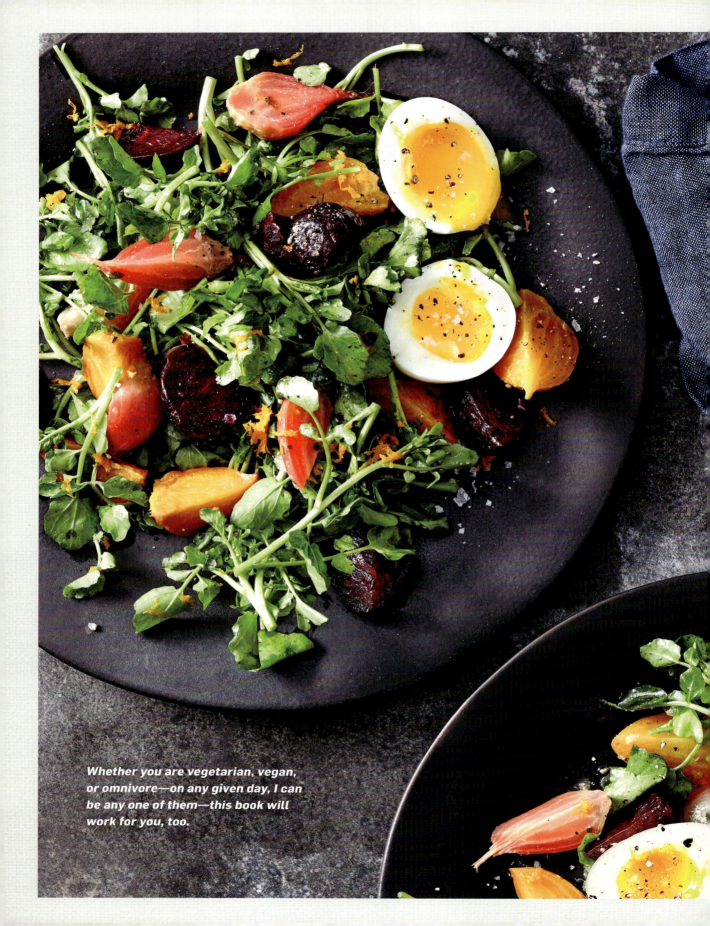

Whether you are vegetarian, vegan, or omnivore—on any given day, I can be any one of them—this book will work for you, too.

introduction

Healthy eating every day is easy when you cook with the right ingredients, including fresh fruits and vegetables in season, locally grown beans and grains, eggs from hens running around outside, and humanely raised meat and poultry. Even where I live, in New York City, I find all of them at our year-round farmers' markets and increasingly at grocery stores that seek out organic food growers and producers who care about quality and sustainability.

I was lucky that my mother understood how closely health and eating were linked long before "wellness" and "holistic" were buzzwords. She didn't call them superfoods, but we ate a diet supercharged with nutrients and micronutrients—whole-grain bread, maple syrup and honey in place of white sugar, and kale decades before it became the poster child for goodness. Turn to page 8 to start reading about how eating fruits and vegetables, smart proteins, good fats, and herbs and spices benefits us. The recipes that follow make eating them every day easy and enticing.

Colorful, boldly flavored dishes can satisfy enough to help you eat moderately. My way of making them is by using flavorful ingredients from all over the world— like miso, Spanish smoked paprika, tahini—that also are rich in phytonutrients and other elements that support optimal wellness.

Eating healthy doesn't have to mean sacrificing pleasure. Indulging a sweet tooth in moderation is essential for me. It means following up a veggie-rich meal with an oat milk-based dark chocolate pudding or spiced grilled peaches. I sometimes crave comfort food, too, so in this book you'll find my deliciously virtuous versions of whole-wheat waffles (made with whole-wheat flour), meatloaf (featuring turkey, plus a savory mushroom gravy), and mashed potatoes (with olive oil swapping in for butter).

Eating healthy includes caring about the earth. For deciding when organic is essential, for fruits and vegetables I follow the Environmental Working Group's Dirty Dozen and Clean Fifteen. When buying meat, I confirm that animals are raised conscientiously. For sustainably harvested seafood, the Monterey Bay Aquarium Seafood Watch has a good guide. I buy at local farmers' markets as much as possible, and bring my reusable bags.

Eating healthy every day includes skipping stress. So along with using super ingredients, let the recipes in *Everyday Healthy* help cooking be a nurturing meditation you enjoy!

Dana Jacobi

The majority of the recipes in this book are meatless, and plenty of dishes are gluten- or dairy-free. Making a recipe fit how you eat is as easy as changing chicken to vegetable broth or making vegan pesto by replacing Parmesan cheese with a non-dairy version. I'll also turn side dishes like Baby Bok Choy, Shiitake Mushroom & Sugar Snap Pea Stir-Fry (page 128) into mains by adding tofu, beef, shrimp, or chicken for protein.

good food for good health

The path to healthy eating begins with choosing whole foods rich in macronutrients and micronutrients. Macronutrients include protein, carbohydrates, and fat. These nutrients allow us to build cells, give us energy, and support our bodies' proper functioning. Micronutrients include the vitamins, minerals, and other compounds we need only in small amounts, which also help our bodies function properly and fight disease.

One group of micronutrients that has garnered attention in recent years is antioxidants. These are vitamins and other substances that boost our immune system and help us repair cells damaged by oxidization—the damaging effects of roving atoms called free radicals that split off from oxygen molecules. Free radicals are created by normal chemical reactions in our bodies, and in lower numbers are actually beneficial to the immune system. However, they become harmful when too many build up within our cells. Aging causes an increase in free radicals, as do air pollution, pesticides, alcohol and tobacco use, and fried foods. An overabundance of free radicals causes inflammation, which in turn is known to cause diseases ranging from arthritis to diabetes to heart disease and cancer. Enter the antioxidants: these substances neutralize free radicals, keeping inflammation in check. Eating a diet rich in antioxidants, therefore, is the best defense against disease and the detrimental effects of aging.

So, healthy eating means including a variety of different foods in our meals, especially a variety of plant-based foods that help us glean many beneficial micronutrients. Nowadays people like to play around with macronutrients: many find that limiting foods like meat, dairy, or refined wheat flour helps them feel less fatigued, which can be a sign of inflammation in the body. If you're feeling out of balance and want to try an adjustment to your usual menu, a key accompanying the recipes in this book shows which recipes are vegan VG, vegetarian V, gluten free GF, or dairy free DF. This will help you try out a macronutrient adjustment and see if it agrees with you! Dishes that include foods especially rich in antioxidants and other micronutrients are given a "superfood" label SF, while dishes that use whole grains—the unrefined carbs that offer slow-release energy and come with their nutrients intact—are flagged WG.

The recipes in this book are meant to be flexible and adjustable. Changing a recipe to fit to how you want to eat can be as easy as changing chicken broth to vegetable broth or making pesto vegan by replacing the Parmesan cheese with a non-dairy version. Or, you can always turn a salad or vegetable side dish into a healthy and satisfying entrée by accompanying it with a poached egg, sautéed chicken breast, broiled fish fillet, or seared tofu.

Read on for more details about the types of ingredients that appear in this book's recipes and the nutrition they offer. Once you understand the role each kind of food plays, you'll be able to choose which recipes suit your current needs, as well as to create your own healthy dishes.

The goal of Everyday Healthy cooking is to offer super-powered meals with an abundance of macro- and micronutrients, helping you create your own daily menus and giving your healthy eating exciting and appealing variety.

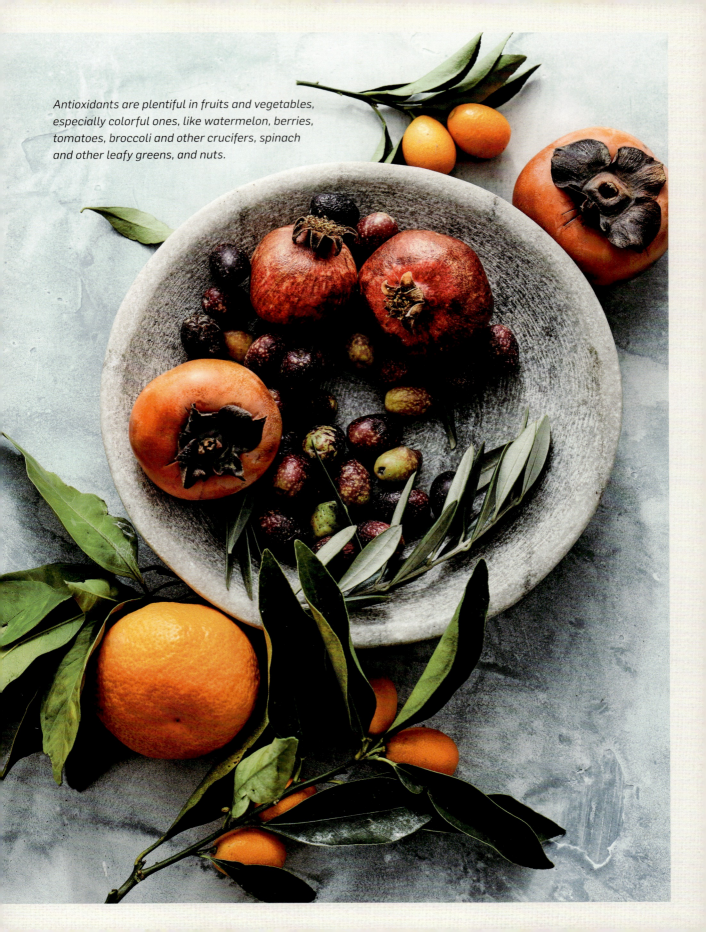

Antioxidants are plentiful in fruits and vegetables, especially colorful ones, like watermelon, berries, tomatoes, broccoli and other crucifers, spinach and other leafy greens, and nuts.

goodness from the garden

Loading your plate with fruits and vegetables gives it appealing color and adds welcome variety in flavor and texture. Variety also matters because each fruit or vegetable offers its own unique combination of micronutrients—vitamins, minerals, and phytonutrients, sometimes called phytochemicals, which are specific nutrients found only in plants that play helpful roles in warding off disease. Some of the most well-known phytonutrients are carotenoids, found in carrots, red berries, and spinach, and polyphenols, found in green tea, soy, and oranges. When buying fresh vegetables and fruits, concentrate on peak-of-season produce grown locally, organic when you can. Choosing local, seasonal ingredients means more nutrients for you and less wear-and-tear on the environment.

VEGETABLES

Vegetables contain a veritable alphabet of phytonutrients. Many are inflammation-fighting antioxidants that specially target a particular health risk, like protecting your vision, fighting the risk of prostate cancer, or reducing the odds of heart disease. Vegetables also offer a wide variety of minerals and vitamins, plus healthy complex carbs for energy, along with filling fiber. Some types, including potatoes, corn, crucifers, and leafy greens, also contain a dose of protein.

CRUCIFERS are a broad family of vegetable powerhouses that includes broccoli, broccoli rabe, Brussels sprouts, bok choy, cabbages, cauliflower, collard greens, and kale. Surprisingly, even arugula, watercress, radishes, and turnips are part of this extended family. The compounds called glucosinolates in cruciferous vegetables are known to have anticancer effects. Each crucifer brings its own blend of vitamins, minerals, and phytonutrients to your table. Many different crucifers appear in recipes throughout this book, helping you eat at least one every day.

LEAFY GREENS include spinach and lettuce, and leafy crucifers like kale, collard greens, arugula, and watercress. Spinach is rich in folate, a B vitamin that protects the heart and protects against birth defects, and is a good source of

iron, which supports energy. Lettuces provide vitamins A, C, and K, plus chromium, a micronutrient that helps maintain stable blood sugar levels.

ROOTS are colorful and rich in complex carbohydrates and fiber. They often contain enough sugar to please your sweet tooth, especially when roasted. The beets in recipes like Roasted Beets wth Indian Spices (page 126) offer unique red antioxidant pigments. Beta-carotene in carrots helps repair damaged DNA in the body, a nice thought while enjoying Carrot Noodles with Kale Pesto (page 134). A trio of carotenoids in orange sweet potatoes can help your immune system resist viruses, so think of Baked Sweet Potatoes with Chili-Lime Butter (page 141) when you feel a cold coming on.

ALLIUMS include onions, green onions, garlic, leeks, and shallots and all contain sulfur-based compounds that help control blood pressure and improve blood cholesterol levels. Yellow onions add the antioxidant quercetin, and red onions add anthocyanins for vision and neurological health. So many dishes use one or more alliums, cooked or raw, that including them in everyday cooking is easy. They even star in Roasted Tomato & Onion Soup (page 36).

VEGETABLE FRUITS

We call the ingredients that follow "vegetables" because of the ways we use them. But botanically speaking, all of them are fruits.

AVOCADOS are one of the most nutrient-dense vegetables. Their mostly monounsaturated fat and beta-sitosterol, a phytonutrient, help balance blood cholesterol levels. Avocados show their culinary versatility in Chocolate Avocado Mousse with Coconut Cream (page 166).

BELL PEPPERS provide good amounts of vitamins A and C. Ripe yellow, red, and orange ones contain the most, while unripe green peppers have the least. Each type of pepper gets its color from different combinations of antioxidant carotenoids. Bell peppers are part of the capsicum family that also includes chiles, but contain no capsaicin, the compound that gives chile peppers their heat. Smoky Black Bean Soup (page 42) showcases the flavor roasted bell peppers add to dishes.

TOMATOES are rich in lycopene, a particularly potent form of carotene that helps protect against heart disease and reduces the risk of prostate, lung, and other cancers. Cooking tomatoes makes it easier for our bodies to utilize their lycopene. Heirloom tomatoes, old-fashioned varieties that were bred more for flavor than for ease of shipping and storage, show off the unique personalities of each variety of this beloved nightshade family. Ripen tomatoes on the counter; do not refrigerate.

FRUITS

The natural sugar in fruit is a better way to satisfy your sweet tooth. Fiber in fruit helps you absorb the sugar more slowly, so your blood sugar spikes less. The pigments that give fruits their vibrant colors also happen to be potent antioxidants. Along with serving fruits in desserts and for snacks, they can go well in savory dishes like Pan-Seared Scallops with Sautéed Citrus (page 85) and Cider-Braised Pork Tenderloin with Roasted Figs (page 108).

APPLES come in numerous varieties and are rich in an array of antioxidants, from vitamin C to quercetin, a very useful anti-inflammatory. They also contain pectin, a form of soluble fiber that helps reduce blood cholesterol. Apples are good in savory dishes, particularly with pork and root vegetables, as well as in desserts and for snacking.

BERRIES are all good sources of fiber. Each kind of berry contains its own unique combination of the antioxidants known as anthocyanins, which also give them their red, blue and purple colors, so enjoy them all, from raspberries, strawberries, and cranberries to blueberries and blackberries. When local berries are out of season, using frozen ones is a good choice. Go organic whenever you can.

KIWIFRUIT contain even more vitamin C than oranges, plenty of potassium, and a useful amount of fiber. Eating them helps reduce inflammation, regulate blood pressure and blood sugar levels, and lutein, another antioxidant, helps lower the risk of cataracts. Kiwis get sweeter and soften when allowed to sit out at room temperature.

MANGO flesh gets its rich orange color from a variety of antioxidant pigments, including anthocyanins and several kinds of carotene. Their fiber helps protect against type 2 diabetes. Yellow-skinned mangoes are the sweetest varieties. Ripen mangoes on the counter; do not refrigerate. Include them in your Supercharged Kale Smoothie (page 179).

CITRUS FRUITS are rich in antioxidant vitamin C and potassium, which helps keep blood pressure even, plus a huge variety of phytochemicals—an orange contains about 170 different ones. Many overlap, but each kind of citrus has some unique phytochemicals. Citrus peel contains aromatic oils with health benefits, so grate the colorful zest over soups and salads and include some in salad dressings.

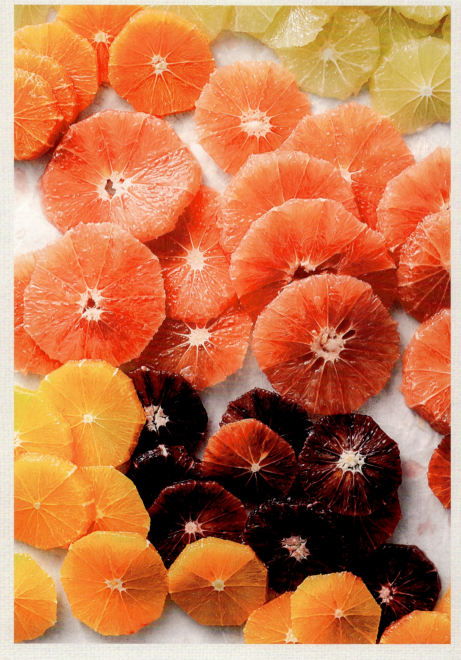

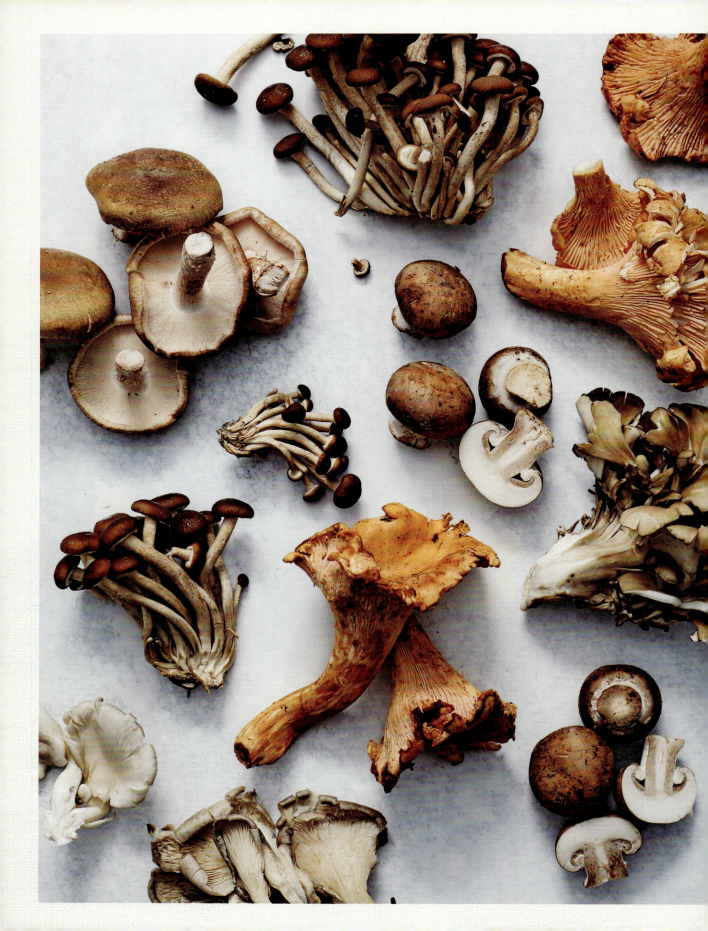

protein power

Every cell in our bodies needs protein. Its amino acids help build and maintain muscle, strengthen bones, repair damaged DNA, and more. Animal protein, containing all nine essential amino acids, is complete. Vegans can benefit from foods with complementary amino acids that together provide the essential nine. Vegetarians can get complete protein by including some cheese, eggs, or dairy in meals.

Some animal foods eaten for protein—including salmon and other oily fish, pastured chicken and chicken eggs, and grass-fed beef—also provide fatty acids such as omega-3s. Important inflammation fighters, omega-3s are necessary in our diet because our bodies cannot make them. Certain plant seeds, such as chia and flax, supply one type of omega-3s. Nuts are also a good source.

FISH & SEAFOOD

The omega-3 fats in fish and seafood help keep our memories sharp and our moods bright. Their anti-inflammatory benefits also help protect us from stroke and improve "good" HDL blood cholesterol. Oily fish, including salmon, sardines, albacore tuna, and mackerel are richest in omega-3s. Cod, trout, halibut, shrimp, and mussels are other good sources. All fish are a super source of vitamin D, which is needed for strong bones and a robust immune system; riboflavin (vitamin B-2), which helps cells function; and zinc, a trace mineral essential for a healthy immune system. Eating fish twice a week is often recommended for optimum health.

MEAT & POULTRY

To bring meat and poultry into your diet in the healthiest way, look for beef, pork, lamb, chicken, and turkey that is raised organically and humanely. "Organic" means animals are given feed or grazed on land entirely without chemical pesticides or fertilizer, raised without hormones or antibiotics, and given outdoor access. Meat from livestock that are grass fed or pastured and poultry that are free-range contains higher amounts of healthy omega-3 fatty acids, so opt for these when possible.

DAIRY

Dairy foods are great sources of protein, calcium, and an abundance of other nutrients, vitamins, and minerals. Their many forms and the complex flavors in cheese and other fermented dairy foods easily add variety to meals. Dairy foods with live cultures, like yogurt and kefir, also contribute greatly to our digestive and immune health.

EGGS

Eggs provide top-quality protein, plus vitamins D and E, choline for brain and eye health, carotenes (a key antioxidant), and potassium, which supports good blood pressure, cardiovascular health, bone strength, and muscle strength. They also contain cholesterol, which is essential to good health but detrimental in overabundance. Unless your body is cholesterol sensitive or insulin resistant, daily eggs are now considered to be a great addition to a healthy diet. Look for organic eggs, preferably from pasture-raised chickens for the highest levels of omega-3s and vitamins A and D.

BEANS & LENTILS

A main source of protein in many cultures, fiber-rich beans and lentils promote a healthy gut and stable blood sugar levels. Each kind of legume has its own personality and combination of antioxidants. Black beans are rich in an antioxidant called kaempferol, thought to help prevent cancer. Lentils are loaded with folate, a B vitamin that helps reduce the risk of birth defects and breaks down homocystine, associated at high levels with depression. Look for locally grown beans, dried or fresh in season. Canned beans are nutritionally as good as dried and a perfect time-saver.

MUSHROOMS

In a class of their own, these edible fungi offer good-quality protein useful in meatless meals. Mushrooms are rich in selenium, a mineral that reduces inflammation and boosts the immune system. Shiitakes are particularly beneficial. All mushrooms, cultivated and wild, add savory umami flavor and a "meaty" feel to dishes.

SOY FOODS

Soybeans are the vegetarian protein champion, providing complete, cholesterol-free protein in a wide variety of forms. Isoflavones, a plant form of estrogen in soy, help protect against osteoporosis and can help relieve the discomforts of menopause. Recipes in this book use traditional soy foods enjoyed for centuries in Asia: tofu, edamame, miso, and tamari.

other healthy ingredients

FIELDS OF GRAIN

Whole grains are important for providing complex carbohydrates, fiber, and even protein, making them especially valuable for meatless meals. They are generally high in iron, magnesium, manganese, phosphorus, selenium, and B vitamins. Whole grains are so called because they still have all the parts nature gave them: the bran, or nutritious outer layer; the germ, or nutrient-rich embryo of the seed; and the endosperm, the germ's energy-rich food supply. Simply switching to eating whole grains in place of refined reduces the risk of diabetes, heart disease, stroke, and various cancers. Whole grains provide a welcome feeling of fullness. Their complex carbs enter the bloodstream more slowly than refined carbs, reducing blood sugar spikes. Fiber helps slow this absorption, too. Buying organic grains assures they are not grown using toxic chemicals. Recipes that make use of whole grains are noted in this book with a (WG) icon, and more details on barley, bulgur, farro, oats, polenta, and quinoa can be found on pages 188–191.

HERBS & SPICES

The recipes in this book aim to get you cooking liberally with herbs and spices whenever possible. Whether you grow them at home or buy them at the store, fresh herbs are worth the effort for the freshness and flavor they bring to healthy cooking. And, you probably guessed it: herbs get their fragrance, flavor, and proven health benefits from phytochemicals and volatile essential oils. Their health-promoting characteristics in clinical tests encourage the liberal use of both fresh and dried herbs.

As for spices, it's a kind of miracle that the warm, room-filling fragrance and vibrant color of spices also come from antioxidant pigments and volatile oils with superpower health benefits. To enjoy and benefit from them most, buy ground spices in the smallest amount you can, as they lose flavor, fragrance, and nutrition quickly, even within months. Consider using a spice grinder to make your own freshly ground spices and bring out their flavor. Turn to pages 188–191 for details on the healthy side of specific herbs and spices.

FERMENTED FOODS

Fermentation breaks down the sugars and carbohydrates in cabbage in kimchi or soybeans in miso, making them easier to digest. This process also makes kimchi taste bold and tangy, and miso savory and umami-rich. The live bacteria in fermented foods join with the good microorganisms in your gut to strengthen your digestive and immune systems. These bacteria are heat-sensitive, so you benefit most when they are not cooked or when they are added towards the end in cooking and heated below boiling point. Yogurt and sauerkraut are other naturally fermented foods rich in beneficial live bacteria.

NUTS & SEEDS

The mono- and polyunsaturated fats in nuts and seeds make eating them good for your heart and brain health by helping to reduce the inflammation associated with heart disease and stroke. Nuts are also a source of plant stanols that help reduce "bad" LDL cholesterol. They contain a useful amount of protein and fiber that helps you feel satisfied. Long-term studies have found that people who snack on a few nuts every day tend to live longer. Nut and seed oils provide some of the same benefits as the whole nut. For details on nut and seed powerhouses like almonds, chia seeds, flax seeds, hemp seeds, pumpkin seeds, sesame seeds, and walnuts, turn to pages 188–191.

HEALTHY OILS

The cooking fats used in this book, mainly olive oil and avocado oil, are high in anti-inflammatory fatty acids and low in saturated fat. Both consist mainly of heart-healthy oleic acid, a monounsaturated omega-9 fatty acid. Avocado oil is less well known than olive oil, but it's great for high-heat cooking and has been found to have beneficial effects on cholesterol levels. Extra-virgin olive oil is full of phenolic antioxidants and adds delicious flavor to uncooked and cooked dishes. For high-heat cooking, both olive oil and avocado oil are resistant to breaking down and oxidizing, compared to a poly-unsaturated fat like canola or soybean oil. More details on avocado oil, coconut oil, olive oil, and grapeseed oil can be found on pages 188–191.

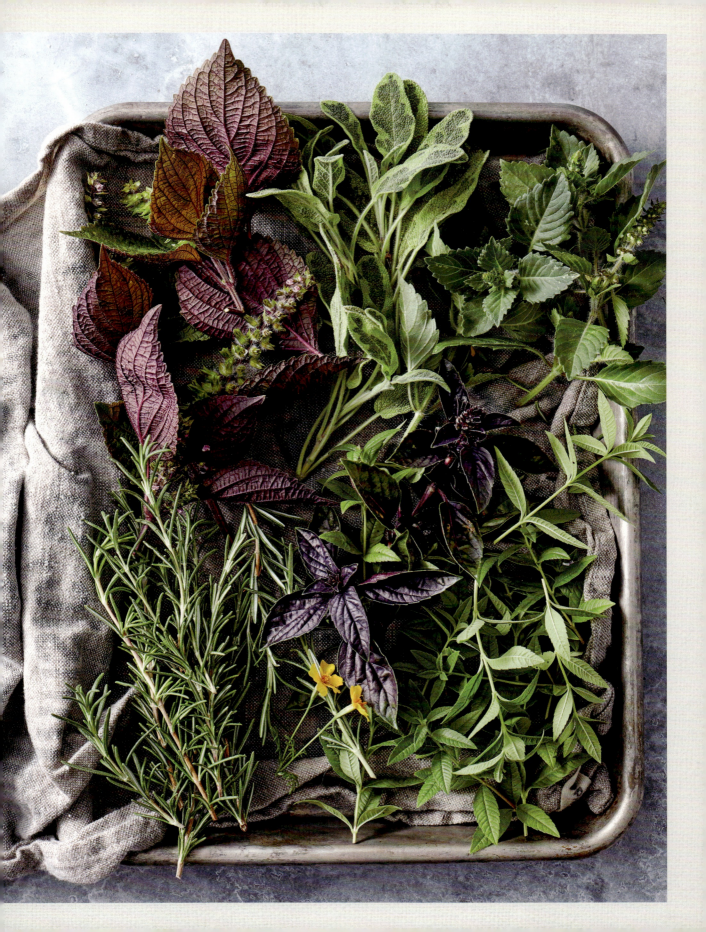

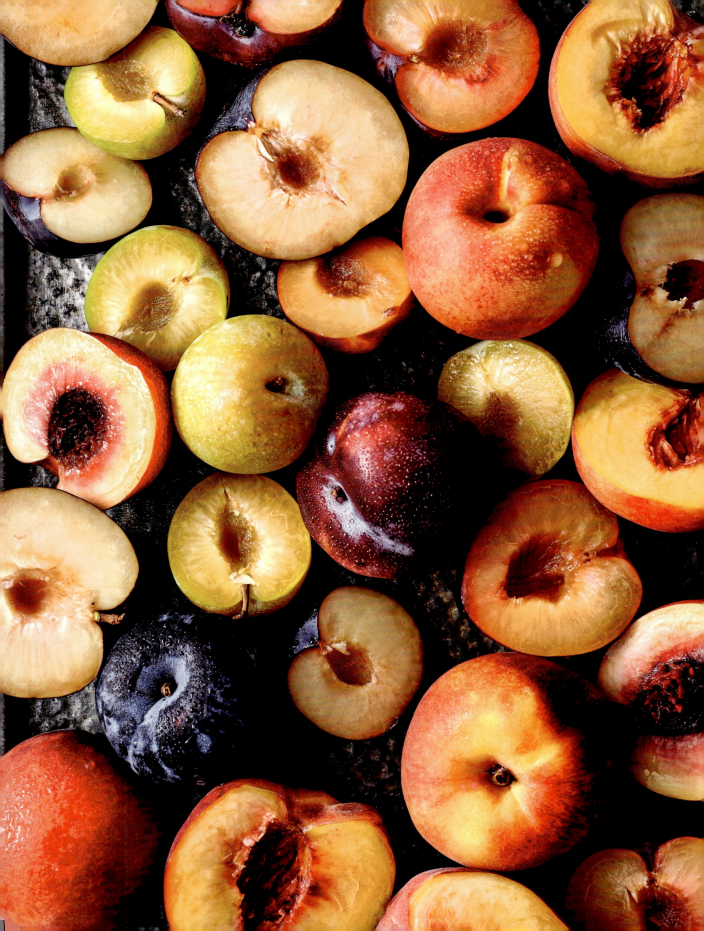

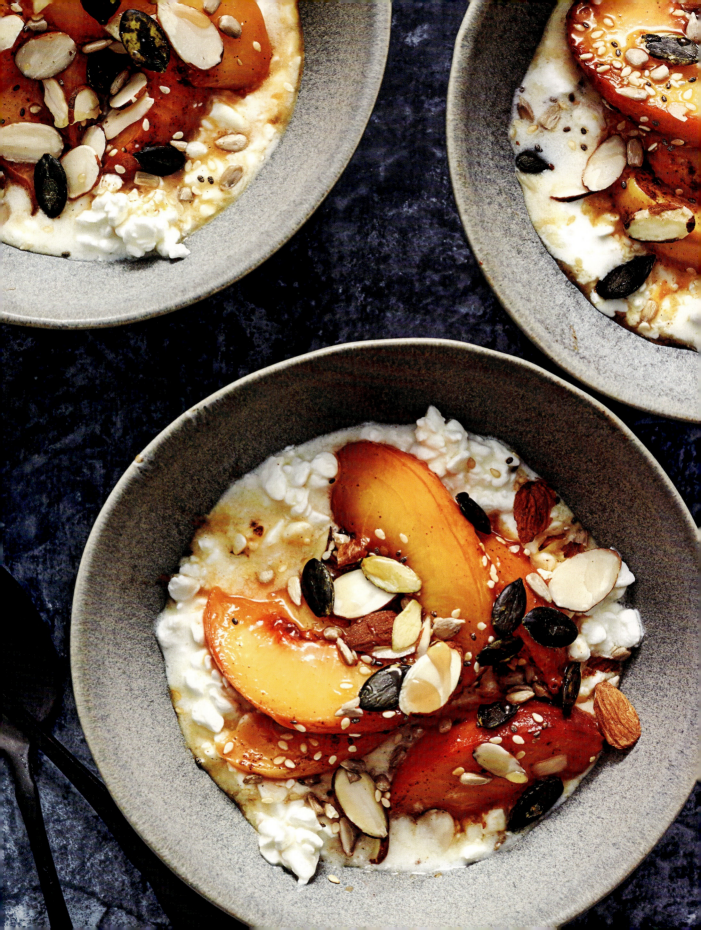

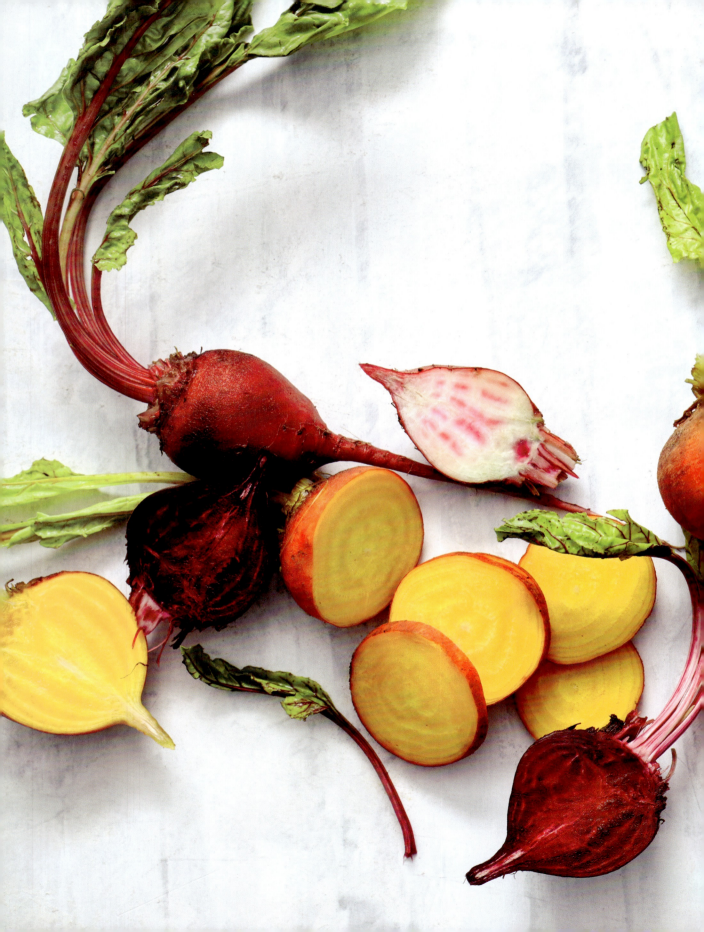

starters & soups

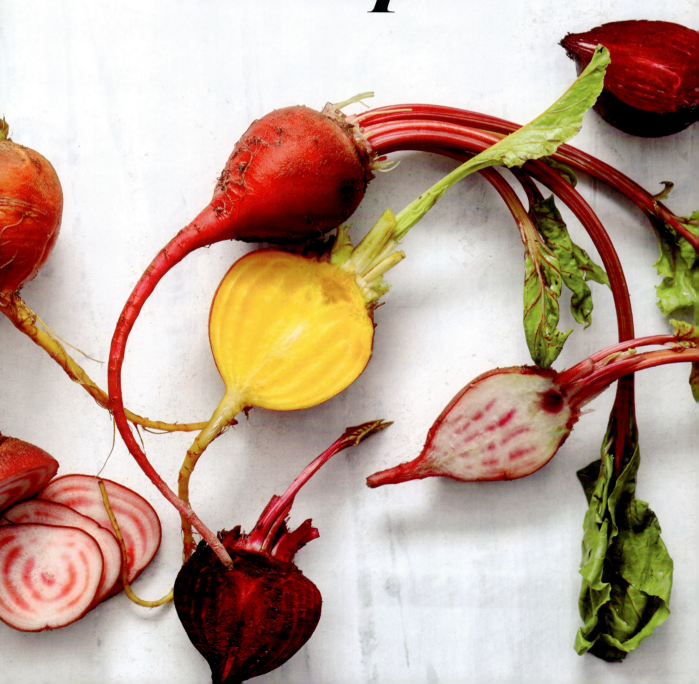

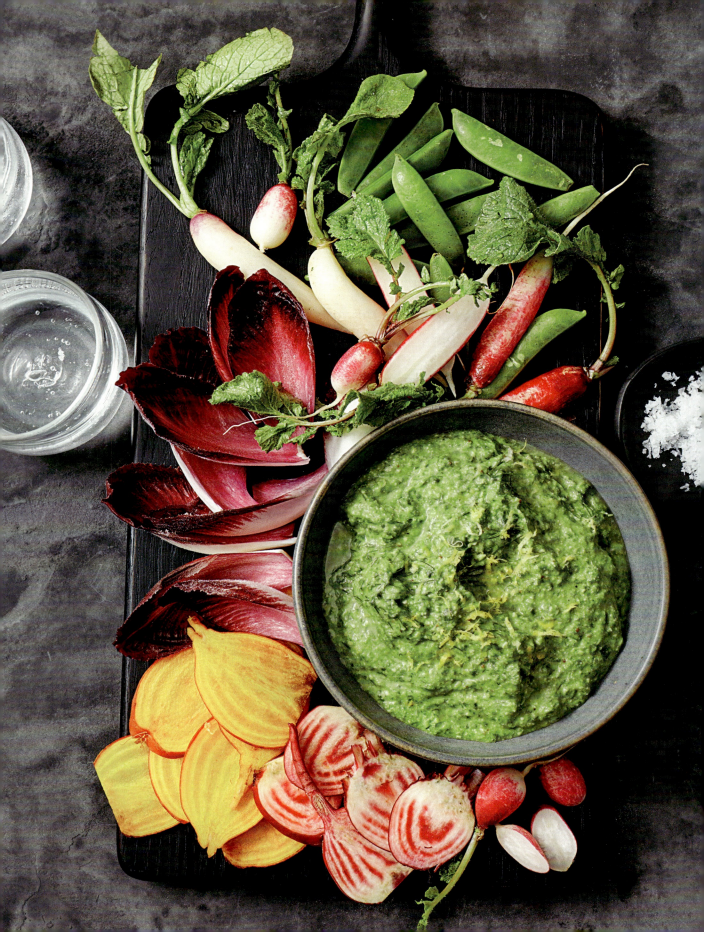

Spinach & Feta Dip with Horseradish

This zesty dip will be your party go-to and a favorite everyday snack, too. Along with bold flavor, the feta brings protein, mayonnaise contributes olive oil's goodness, and lemon juice contains acid that helps your body access more of the iron in the spinach. Together with the horseradish's kick, they give this full-bodied dip maximum health benefits along with great taste.

4 SERVINGS
(ABOUT 1¼ CUPS/300 ML)

4 oz (120 g) raw baby spinach (4 packed cups)

½ cup (2 oz/60 g) crumbled feta cheese

2 green onions, white and pale green parts, roughly chopped

¼ cup (60 ml) olive-oil mayonnaise

1 Tbsp whole-grain mustard

1 tsp fresh lemon juice

¼ cup (15 g) chopped fresh dill, plus sprigs for garnish

Sea salt and freshly ground black pepper

Baby carrots, celery sticks, radishes, sugar snap peas, endive leaves, and/or multicolor bell pepper strips, for serving

In a food processor, pulse the spinach until finely chopped. Add the feta and green onions and pulse to combine them with the spinach. Add the mayonnaise, mustard, and lemon juice and whirl until mixture is a textured purée. Add the chopped dill and pulse just to blend. Thanks to the feta, the dip may need little or no salt, but season it liberally with pepper. Scoop the dip into a serving bowl. Garnish with the dill sprigs and serve right away, accompanied by the vegetables of your choice.

Smoky Roasted Eggplant Dip with Cumin-Crusted Pita

An ideal appetizer or snack, this dip is a delicious way to add fiber to your diet. Tahini, along with contributing nutty richness, is a good source of calcium. Think of this appealingly smoky dip especially from July through October, when locally grown eggplant are in season.

8 SERVINGS

FOR THE PITA CHIPS

1 tsp cumin seeds

¾ tsp kosher salt

3 pita breads, 7 inches (18 cm) in diameter

1 ½ Tbsp olive oil

FOR THE DIP

6 cloves garlic, unpeeled, ends trimmed

1 tsp olive oil, plus more for greasing

2 globe eggplants (about 2 lb/1 kg total weight), halved lengthwise

2 Tbsp fresh lemon juice

¼ cup (60 g) tahini

Sea salt

¼ tsp smoked paprika

Preheat the oven to 400°F (200°C). Line a rimmed baking sheet with aluminum foil.

To make the pita chips, in a small frying pan over medium heat, toast the cumin seeds, stirring frequently, until fragrant, about 2 minutes. Pour onto a plate to cool. Transfer the cumin seeds to a spice mill or mortar, add the salt, and grind or crush with a pestle until finely ground.

Brush the pita breads on both sides with the olive oil, cut each into 8 wedges, and arrange them on the prepared baking sheet. Sprinkle the tops evenly with the cumin mixture. Bake until the wedges are light golden brown and crisp, 10–15 minutes, turning them over halfway through baking. Set aside.

To make the eggplant dip, place the cloves on a small square of aluminum foil, drizzle with the 1 tsp olive oil, and wrap securely in the foil. Place on the same pan and bake until the garlic is soft, about 15 minutes. Unwrap and let stand until cool enough to handle.

Preheat the broiler. Line a broiler pan with aluminum foil and lightly grease with oil. Place the eggplants on the prepared pan, cut-side down, and broil until the skins char and the flesh is tender, about 20 minutes. Transfer the eggplant to a colander and set it in the sink to drain and cool slightly.

Using a spoon, scrape the eggplant flesh out of the skins into a blender. Squeeze the roasted garlic from its skins and add to the blender along with the lemon juice, tahini, and a pinch of salt. Blend the ingredients until smooth, and then taste and season with additional salt. Transfer the dip to a serving bowl and let stand for a few minutes to allow the flavors to blend. Sprinkle the dip with the paprika and place on a platter. Arrange the pita chips alongside and serve.

Red Lentil Dip with Smoked Paprika & Rainbow Veggie Dippers

Serve this powerhouse Mediterranean dip with crudités to nosh on while dinner is being prepared, or as a light meal. Creamy red lentils cook in twenty minutes and provide protein and fiber. Walnuts bring heart-healthy omega-3 fat and cancer-fighting antioxidants. Even the spices add important micronutrients.

4 SERVINGS
(ABOUT 1¼ CUPS/300 ML)

⅓ cup (70 g) dried red lentils

2 Tbsp olive oil

½ cup (60 g) chopped yellow onion

1 large clove garlic, chopped

½ tsp ground cumin

¼ tsp smoked paprika

⅓ cup (40 g) walnuts, coarsely chopped

⅓ cup (60 g) coarsely chopped roasted red bell pepper (see Tip)

1 tsp fresh lime juice

Sea salt and freshly ground black pepper

FOR DIPPERS

2 cups (180 g) bite-sized broccoli florets

1 red bell pepper, seeded and cut in strips

1 yellow bell pepper, seeded and cut in strips

1 large carrot, cut into 3-inch (7.5-cm) sticks

In a medium bowl, cover the lentils with cold water to a depth of 2 inches (5 cm). Swish with your hand, then drain the lentils. Repeat 3 or 4 times, until the drained water runs almost clear.

Put the lentils in a medium saucepan and add 1¼ cups (300 ml) water. Bring to a boil over high heat, reduce the heat to low, cover partially, and simmer until very soft, 20 minutes. Set aside.

In a medium frying pan over medium-high heat, heat the oil. Add the onion and cook, stirring occasionally, until softened, about 4 minutes. Add the garlic and cook, stirring occasionally, until the onions are very soft, 3 minutes longer. Mix in the cumin and smoked paprika and cook until fragrant, about 30 seconds. Scrape the onion mixture into a food processor. Add the walnuts and pulse until you have a pulpy purée. Add the lentils, roasted peppers, and lime juice and process until the dip is almost smooth. Season with salt and pepper to taste.

Place the dip in a serving bowl, set on a serving platter, and surround with broccoli florets, red and yellow bell pepper strips, and carrot sticks. Serve right away.

TIP *Jarred roasted red peppers are an excellent time-saving ingredient to keep on hand in the pantry cupboard at all times.*

Crostini with Whipped Goat Cheese, Roasted Grapes & Rosemary

Goat cheese is lower in lactose than other cheeses and marries beautifully with the earthiness of rosemary. Roasting the grapes deepens their flavor and sweetness, which comes from natural sugars that contribute healthy minerals and nutrients stripped away during the chemical processing of granulated sugar and corn syrup.

8–10 SERVINGS

**48 thin slices baguette
(about ¾ baguette)**

**7 Tbsp (100 ml) extra-virgin
olive oil**

**Kosher salt and freshly ground
black pepper**

**1 lb (500 g) seedless red grapes,
separated into small bunches**

**3 fresh rosemary sprigs,
plus 2 Tbsp minced leaves**

**½ lb (250 g) goat cheese,
at room temperature**

3 Tbsp whole milk

Honey, for drizzling

Flaky sea salt, for finishing

Preheat the oven to 350°F (180°C). On a large baking sheet, arrange the baguette slices in a single layer. Brush the tops of the slices with 5 Tbsp (75 ml) of the oil and season generously with kosher salt and pepper. Toast the slices, flipping once halfway through, until the slices are golden, the edges are crisp, and the centers are still slightly soft, about 10 minutes. Let cool completely.

Raise the oven temperature to 425°F (220°C). Arrange the grape bunches and the rosemary sprigs on a second baking sheet. Drizzle with 1 tablespoon of the oil and season with kosher salt. Roast until the grapes are soft, have shriveled a bit, and are beginning to burst, about 15 minutes. Let cool.

In a stand mixer fitted with the whisk attachment, combine the goat cheese, the remaining 1 tablespoon oil, and the milk and beat on high speed until light and fluffy, about 3 minutes. Stir in the minced rosemary.

To serve, spread each bread slice with some of the cheese, top with a few roasted grapes, and drizzle with a little honey. Finish with a light dusting of sea salt, and serve.

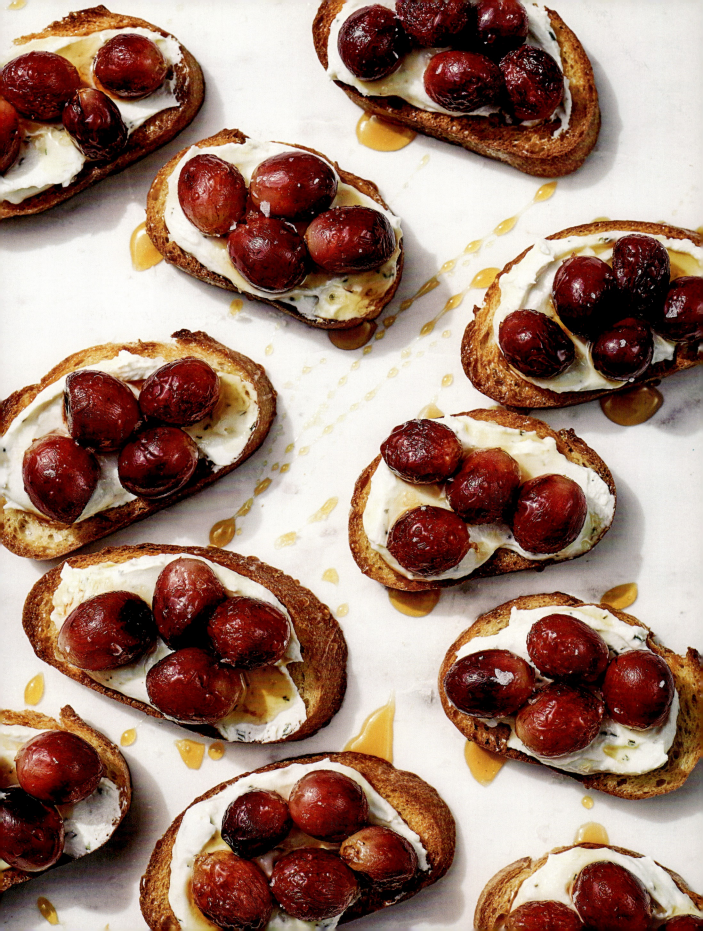

Chickpea & Hemp Seed Hummus with Roasted Garlic

Hemp seeds give this classic chickpea hummus a nutritional boost by adding healthy omega-3 fat, and they also make its texture super creamy. Roasted garlic gives it softer pungency than using raw cloves. To turn this hummus into a nice nutrient-dense dressing to drizzle over a salad of romaine lettuce, watercress, and grape tomatoes, simply thin it with a little more water.

8 SERVINGS

1 can (15.5 oz/439 g) chickpeas, drained and rinsed

2 Tbsp shelled hemp seeds

¼ cup (60 g) roasted tahini

4 cloves roasted garlic

2 tsp ground cumin

¼ cup (60 ml) fresh lemon juice

¼ cup (60 ml) warm water

¼ cup (60 ml) extra-virgin olive oil

Sea salt

Chopped fresh flat-leaf parsley, Kalamata olives, and/or cayenne pepper, for serving (optional)

Whole-wheat pita breads cut into wedges

In a food processor, combine the chickpeas and hemp seeds and pulse until coarsely chopped. Add the tahini, garlic, cumin, lemon juice, water, and olive oil and whirl until the mixture is creamy. Season to taste with salt. Transfer the hummus to a serving bowl, cover, and refrigerate for 30 minutes to let flavors meld. Serve garnished with parsley, olives, and/or a dash of cayenne, if desired, and accompanied by pita bread wedges. The hummus will keep covered in the refrigerator for up to 5 days.

Wild Mushroom Flatbread with Fontina & Thyme

The flavorful topping of this satisfying flatbread is enhanced by sautéing the mushrooms with thyme and a touch of wine. Mozzarella made from water buffalo milk is virtually lactose-free while part- and skim milk cow's milk versions contain substantially less lactose. If using fresh mozzarella, slice it thinly and let it dry on paper towels for 30 minutes to avoid making the flatbread soggy.

**2 FLATBREADS;
4 SERVINGS**

3 Tbsp olive oil, plus more for brushing

2 shallots, minced

2 cloves garlic, minced

1 lb (500 g) mixed fresh mushrooms such as chanterelle, black trumpet, hedgehog, and cremini, brushed clean, tough stems trimmed, and roughly chopped

2 Tbsp unsalted butter

½ cup (125 ml) dry white wine

3 fresh thyme or other herb sprigs, plus leaves for garnish

Kosher salt and freshly ground black pepper

All-purpose flour, for dusting

¾ lb (350 g) pizza dough, homemade (page 189) or store-bought, at room temperature

1 cup (4 oz/120 g) shredded Fontina cheese

1 cup (4 oz/120 g) shredded mozzarella cheese

Flaky sea salt, for finishing

Position a rack in the upper third of the oven and place a pizza stone or an oiled upside-down baking sheet on the rack. Preheat the oven to 450°F (230°C).

In a large frying pan over medium-high heat, heat the oil. Add the shallots and garlic and cook, stirring often, until the shallots are softened, about 3 minutes. Add the mushrooms and continue to cook, stirring occasionally, until the mushrooms are lightly browned, about 5 minutes. Add the butter, wine, and thyme sprigs, reduce the heat to medium-low, and cook, stirring occasionally, until the mushrooms are caramelized and the wine is completely absorbed, about 5 minutes longer. Season to taste with salt and pepper, remove from the heat, discard the thyme sprigs, and set aside.

Place the dough on a lightly floured work surface and divide in half. One at a time, using a rolling pin, roll and stretch each dough portion into an elongated oval about ½ inch (12 mm) thick. Transfer the dough to the stone or baking sheet and bake until lightly golden and beginning to crisp, 6–8 minutes. Carefully remove the flatbreads from the oven and top each one with ½ cup (55 g) each of the Fontina and mozzarella and half of the mushroom mixture. Brush the crust edges with oil and return the flatbreads to the oven until the cheeses have melted and the edges of the crust are golden brown, 8–10 minutes longer.

Transfer to a cutting board and top with flaky salt and thyme leaves. Cut into triangles and serve.

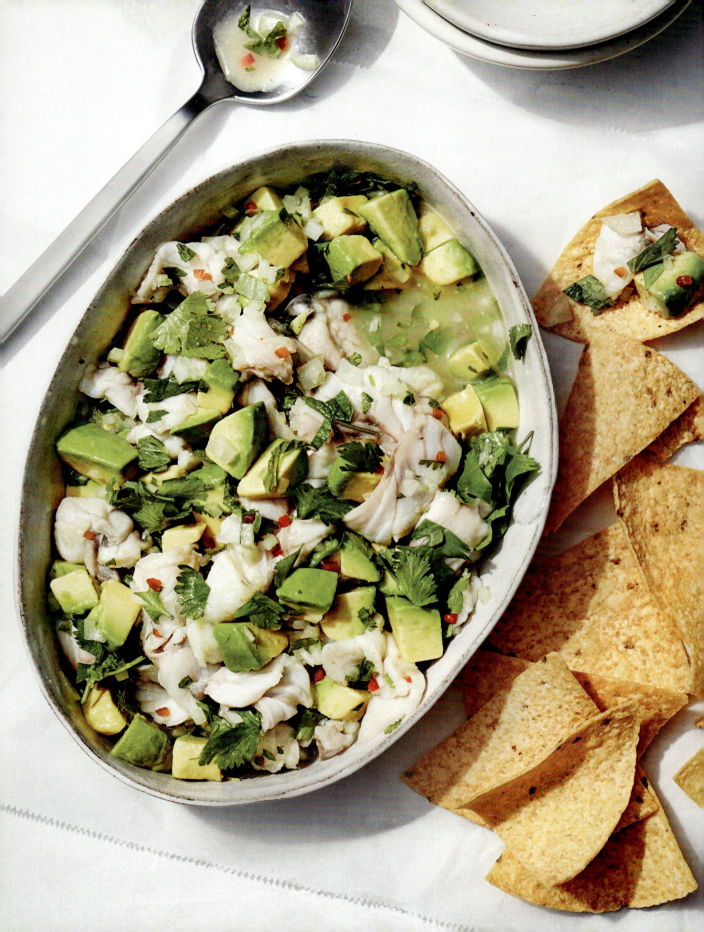

Ceviche with Lime & Herbs

The slightly bitter tang of lime juice is particularly appealing in savory dishes like this easy ceviche as well as in desserts and drinks. The juice has traces of potassium, calcium, and vitamin A but its greatest benefit comes from its powerful punch of vitamin C for which this dish provides about a third of one's daily recommended requirement.

6 SERVINGS

1 lb (500 g) boneless firm white-fleshed fish, such as snapper or halibut, cut into ½-inch (12-mm) pieces

1 ⅓ cups (320 ml) fresh lime juice

¼ cup (45 g) minced white onion

1 red jalapeño chile, minced

1 avocado, halved, pitted, and diced

¼ cup (15 g) chopped fresh cilantro

2 Tbsp finely chopped fresh mint

Sea salt and freshly ground black pepper

Tortilla chips, for serving

In a bowl, stir together the fish pieces, lime juice, onion, and jalapeño. Cover and refrigerate until the fish is opaque throughout, 30–60 minutes.

Using a slotted spoon, transfer the fish, onions, and jalapeño to another bowl, leaving the liquid behind. Stir in the avocado, cilantro, and mint, and season with salt and pepper. Taste, and add some of the marinade if desired for more acidity.

Serve right away with the tortilla chips.

Grilled Shrimp with Green Onions & Romesco

A meal of grilled new-crop spring onions with smoky romesco sauce is an annual tradition in Catalonia. This version of that ritual Spanish meal includes succulent shrimp, providing an added boost of protein that makes for a satisfying starter or light meal. Jarred sweet piquillo peppers for authentic romesco are sold in specialty-food stores and online, but roasted red bell peppers can be substituted.

4 SERVINGS

FOR THE ROMESCO SAUCE

1 jar (about 10 ½ oz/300 g) piquillo peppers, drained

½ cup (70 g) almonds, toasted and chopped

¼ cup (60 ml) extra-virgin olive oil

3 cloves garlic, chopped

2 tsp smoked paprika

Kosher salt and freshly ground black pepper

FOR THE SHRIMP

12 jumbo shrimp, peeled and deveined

¼ cup (60 ml) olive oil

4 cloves garlic, pressed

2 tsp smoked paprika

16 spring onions or green onions

2 lemons, halved crosswise

Prepare a grill for direct-heat cooking over medium heat, or use a stove-top grill pan. Oil the grill grate or pan. To make the romesco sauce, in a blender, combine the piquillo peppers, almonds, olive oil, garlic, and paprika and process until smooth. Pour into a bowl and season with salt. Set aside at room temperature.

In a bowl, combine the shrimp, 2 Tbsp of the olive oil, the garlic, and the paprika and turn to coat the shrimp evenly. Coat the spring onions and lemons lightly with the remaining 2 Tbsp olive oil.

Arrange the shrimp on the grill rack or pan and season with salt and pepper. Cook for about 3 minutes, then add the spring onions and lemons, cut-side down. Cook, turning all the items as needed, until the shrimp are opaque throughout and the spring onions and lemons are lightly charred, about 6 minutes total for the shrimp and 3 minutes total for the spring onions and lemons. Transfer the shrimp, green onions, and lemons to a platter, and serve with the romesco sauce.

Beet-Cured Salmon Platter

Curing salmon with raw beets produces gorgeous fish marbled with rich hues of pink and red, a perfect showstopper dish for entertaining. Leftovers, if you are lucky, are excellent served the next day for a protein-rich weekend post-workout brunch, paired with multigrain bagels and pickled onion. Ideally, have the fishmonger cut the salmon from the plump center portion of a fillet.

8 SERVINGS

3 cups (700 g) coarse kosher salt

3 cups (600 g) sugar

3 lb (1.5 kg) beets, peeled and grated

2 lb (1 kg) skinless salmon fillets

FOR SERVING

2 heads Little Gem lettuce (about 6 oz/175 g total weight), leaves separated

6 oz (180 g) green beans, trimmed, cooked until tender-crisp, and cut into 2-inch (5-cm) lengths

¾ lb (350 g) red potatoes, boiled and cut crosswise into slices ½ inch (12 mm) thick

3 hard-cooked eggs, peeled and cut crosswise into slices ½ inch (12 mm) thick (see Tip)

1 pint (340 g) cherry tomatoes, halved

4 radishes, thinly sliced

1 cup (150 g) Castelvetrano olives, halved lengthwise and pitted

Flaky sea salt and freshly ground black pepper

1 ½ cups (350 ml) Avocado Green Goddess Dressing (page 186)

To make the cured salmon, line a baking sheet with parchment paper. In a bowl, whisk together the salt and sugar, mixing well. Spread half of the beets on the prepared pan in an even layer slightly larger than the salmon. Pour half of the salt mixture over the beets and spread into an even layer to cover. Place the salmon on top of the salt mixture, then cover the salmon evenly with the remaining salt mixture. Spread the remaining beets over the top and pat to pack firmly. Cover the salmon with more parchment and wrap the tray tightly with plastic wrap. Refrigerate for 3 days.

Unwrap the salmon and scrape off and discard the beets and salt mixture. Rinse the salmon under cool running water to remove any last bits of the cure, and pat dry. (At this point, you can wrap the salmon tightly and store in the fridge for up to 1 week.)

To assemble the dish, make a bed of the lettuce leaves on a large platter. Arrange the green beans, potatoes, eggs, tomatoes, radishes, and olives on the lettuce. Thinly slice the salmon against the grain and arrange on the platter. Season the salad with flaky salt and fresh pepper, and serve the dressing on the side.

TIP *To hard-cook eggs, place them in a saucepan with enough water to cover by 1 inch (2.5 cm). Bring to a boil over medium-high heat. Remove the pan from the heat, cover, and let stand until done to your liking, about 10 minutes for slightly runny yolks and up to 14 minutes for firm yolks. Drain the eggs, then transfer to a bowl of ice water to cool slightly, about 2 minutes.*

GF SF

Asian-Style Chicken Soup with Baby Bok Choy

Here, chicken and vegetables are cooked in a clear, spice-infused broth. Served with herbs and bean sprouts, it makes a refreshing one-dish starter or meal packed with protein, fiber, and vitamins C and A. If you do not have a large tea ball, tie the spices in a square of cheesecloth.

4 SERVINGS

8 cups (2 l) low-sodium chicken broth

1 bunch green onions

2-inch (5-cm) piece fresh ginger, peeled and sliced

2 Tbsp Asian fish sauce

1 Tbsp sugar

6 star anise pods

6 cloves

1–1 ¼ lb (500–570 g) boneless, skinless chicken breasts

3 Thai chiles or 1 serrano chile, thinly sliced

Bean sprouts, fresh basil sprigs, fresh cilantro sprigs, and lime wedges, for serving

Hoisin sauce, for serving (optional)

4 baby bok choy

6–7 oz (180–200 g) dried rice stick noodles (maifun)

Coarse kosher salt and freshly ground black pepper

In a large pot over high heat, combine the broth and 2 cups (500 ml) water. Cut the green onion bunch in half crosswise and add the bottom halves to the pot; add the ginger, fish sauce, and sugar. (Thinly slice the green onion tops and reserve.) In a tea ball, combine the star anise and cloves; add to the pot. Bring the broth to a boil. Add the chicken breasts, return to a boil, reduce the heat to medium-low, and simmer until the chicken is cooked through, 10–15 minutes, depending on the size of the breasts. Using tongs, transfer the chicken to a plate and set aside until ready to use. Simmer the broth to develop flavor, 15–30 minutes.

Place the sliced green onions, sliced chiles, bean sprouts, herb sprigs, lime wedges, and hoisin sauce, if using, on a platter or in small bowls, and set out on the table.

Slice the bok choy crosswise about ½ inch (12 mm) thick. Thinly slice the chicken breasts crosswise. Place the noodles in a large heatproof bowl. Cover the noodles with very hot water and let soak for 3 minutes.

Using tongs, remove the green onions and ginger from the pot and discard. Season the broth to taste with salt and pepper. Add the baby bok choy to the pot, raise the heat to high, and bring to a boil. Drain the noodles, add to the broth, and cook until just tender, about 2 minutes.

Using tongs, divide the noodles and bok choy among deep bowls. Divide the chicken among the bowls. Ladle the broth over the top. Serve right away, passing the condiments at the table.

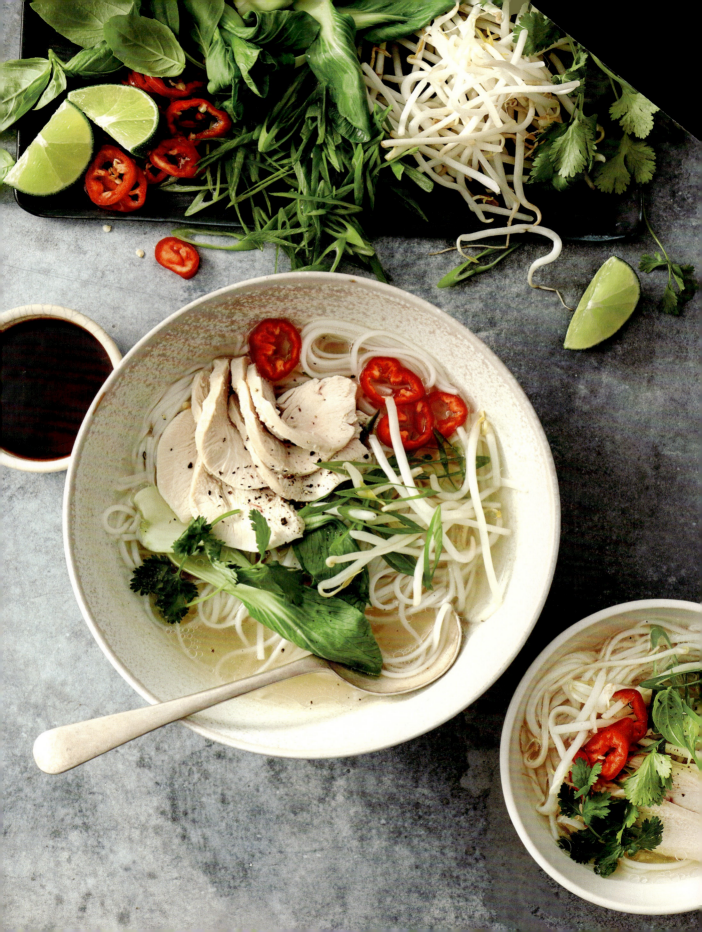

Roasted Beet Soup with Dill & Feta

Once thought of as humble, unglamorous kitchen staples, beets—containing a wealth of minerals and boasting anti-inflammatory properties—offer an appealing deep, rich red color combined with a sweet, earthy flavor and tender texture. Don't let the cheese scare you away—besides creating a beautiful color contrast, feta is low in lactose and digestible even for the lactose-intolerant.

4 SERVINGS

3 large beets, trimmed leaving 1 inch (2.5 cm) of stem

1 ½ Tbsp olive oil

1 Tbsp unsalted butter

¼ cup (40 g) diced yellow onion

4 cups (1 l) low-sodium beef or vegetable broth

Sea salt and freshly ground black pepper

½ cup (2 oz/60 g) crumbled feta cheese

1 Tbsp dill, coarsely chopped

Preheat the oven to 350°F (180°C). Put the beets in a baking dish and drizzle evenly with the olive oil, turning them to coat well. Roast until tender when pierced with a fork, about 1 hour, depending on their size.

Remove from the oven. When cool, peel the beets and coarsely chop. Set aside.

In a large saucepan over medium heat, melt the butter. Add the onion and sauté until translucent, about 2 minutes. Add the chopped beets and the broth and bring to a simmer. Reduce the heat to low and cook, uncovered, for about 10 minutes.

Using an immersion blender, purée the soup. (Alternatively, transfer the soup in batches to a stand blender and process until smooth.) Return the soup to medium heat and season with salt and pepper. Reheat the soup gently just until hot.

Ladle the soup into serving bowls, top with the feta cheese and dill, and serve right away.

English Pea & Watercress Soup

Emerald green and bursting with the bright flavors of peas, watercress, and green onions, this spring soup delivers more than enough of one's daily vitamins and minerals, especially vitamin K. The russet potato gives this soup silky smooth texture without the saturated fat and calories of cream, plus it adds vitamin C.

4–6 SERVINGS

1 Tbsp olive oil

⅔ cup (60 g) sliced green onions, white and pale green parts, plus more for garnish

2 cloves garlic, chopped

1 tsp peeled and grated fresh ginger

5 cups (1.25 l) low-sodium chicken or vegetable broth

1 russet potato (about ½ lb/ 250 g), peeled and cut into 1-inch (2.5-cm) chunks

4 cups (4 oz/120 g) watercress, tough stems removed

3 cups (345 g) English peas, shelled

⅓ cup (80 g) crème fraîche, plus more for garnish

Kosher salt and freshly ground black pepper

In a large, heavy saucepan over medium-high heat, heat the olive oil.

Add the green onions, garlic, and ginger and sauté until the green onions are tender, about 1 minute. Add the broth and potato and bring to a simmer. Reduce the heat to medium, cover, and cook until the potato is very tender, about 12 minutes.

Stir in the watercress and peas, re-cover, and continue to cook until the peas are tender, about 4 minutes. Remove from the heat and let cool slightly.

Using an immersion blender, purée the soup. (Alternatively, transfer the soup in batches to a stand blender and process until smooth.) Return the soup to medium heat and whisk in the crème fraîche. Reheat just until the soup reaches a simmer. Season with salt and pepper. Ladle the soup into bowls, garnish with crème fraîche and green onions, and serve.

Roasted Tomato & Onion Soup

This simple dish blends three powerful superfoods—tomatoes, garlic, and onions—into a silky soup. The tomatoes are first roasted in a medium-hot oven to concentrate their flavors and enhance their sweetness. Use vegetable broth for a vegetarian version of the soup.

4–6 SERVINGS

3 lb (1.5 kg) ripe tomatoes

2 Tbsp olive oil

2 Tbsp balsamic vinegar

1 clove garlic, minced

2 tsp fresh thyme leaves

Sea salt and freshly ground black pepper

1 yellow onion, chopped

½ cup (125 ml) dry white wine

3 cups (700 ml) low-sodium chicken or vegetable broth

2 Tbsp chopped fresh flat-leaf parsley

Preheat the oven to 325°F (165°C). Cut the tomatoes in half and place, cut-side up, on a baking sheet. In a small bowl, whisk together 1 Tbsp of the olive oil, the vinegar, garlic, thyme, ¼ tsp salt, and ¼ tsp pepper. Spoon the mixture evenly over the tomatoes. Roast until the tomatoes are soft and wrinkled, about 1 hour.

In a soup pot over medium-high heat, heat the remaining 1 Tbsp olive oil. Add the onion and cook, stirring often and reducing the heat as necessary to prevent scorching, until soft, 5–7 minutes. Add the wine, raise the heat to medium-high, and bring to a boil. Cook until the liquid is evaporated, 2–3 minutes. Stir in the broth and roasted tomatoes, using a wooden spoon to scrape up any browned bits from the pan, and return to a boil. Reduce the heat to medium-low, cover, and simmer for 10 minutes to allow the flavors to blend.

Using an immersion blender, purée the soup. (Alternatively, transfer the soup in batches to a stand blender and process until smooth.) Return the soup to medium heat and season with salt and pepper. Reheat the soup gently just until hot.

Ladle the soup into serving bowls, garnish with the parsley, and serve right away.

Tuscan-Style Bean & Kale Soup

This rustic soup is packed with super-healthy ingredients. It tastes even better when made a day ahead. If you have leftovers, on the second day, do as the Italians do and ladle the reheated soup into bowls containing a thick slice of stale whole-grain bread.

8 SERVINGS

1 cup (200 g) dried borlotti or cranberry beans

1 bunch Tuscan kale (about ½ lb/250 g)

2 Tbsp olive oil

1 large yellow onion, chopped

1 large carrot, peeled and chopped

1 rib celery, thinly sliced

2 cloves garlic, minced

1 can (28 oz/794 g) whole Roma (plum) tomatoes

1 bay leaf

Pinch of red chile flakes

Sea salt and freshly ground black pepper

Pick over the beans for stones or broken or misshapen beans. Rinse thoroughly under cold running water and drain. Put the beans in a bowl and add fresh water to cover by 3–4 inches (7.5–10 cm). Let soak for at least 4 hours and up to overnight.

Drain the beans and transfer them to a soup pot. Add water to cover the beans generously. Bring to a boil over high heat, reduce the heat to low, cover partially, and simmer gently until the beans are tender, 1–1 ½ hours, depending on the freshness of the beans. Drain the beans, pouring their liquid into another pot or a heatproof bowl. Set aside the beans and liquid separately.

Cut the stems from the kale leaves and discard. Stack the leaves, roll them up lengthwise, and cut crosswise into strips about ½ inch (12 mm) wide.

In a soup pot over medium-high heat, heat the olive oil. Add the onion, carrot, and celery and sauté until the onion is translucent, 5–7 minutes. Add the kale and stir until wilted, about 5 minutes. Add the garlic and sauté until fragrant, about 1 minute. Pour the tomatoes into a bowl and, using your hands, crush them into small pieces. Add the tomatoes and their juices to the pot and stir to combine.

Measure the bean-cooking liquid and add water as needed to total 4 cups (1 l). Add the beans and the cooking-liquid mixture to the pot along with the bay leaf and red chile flakes. Bring to a boil over medium-high heat, reduce the heat to medium-low, cover, and simmer just until the beans are heated through, about 10 minutes. Season to taste with salt and pepper.

Ladle the soup into individual bowls and serve right away.

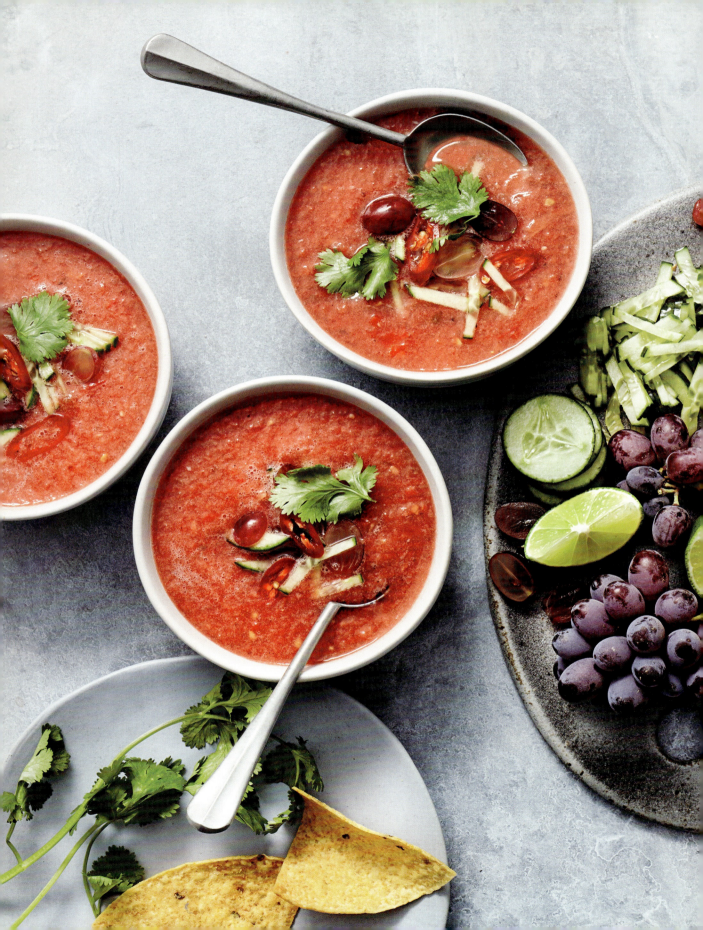

Watermelon Gazpacho

This refreshing soup is as easy to make as whipping up a smoothie. Whirl it up in the morning, then chill it to serve for dinner at the end of a hot day. Watermelon and tomatoes are loaded with antioxidants proven to benefit your eyes, skin, and more. Using your favorite prepared green salsa lets you give it just the amount of heat you like.

4 SERVINGS

3 cups (450 g) cubed seedless watermelon

2 ½ cups (375 g) seeded and cubed ripe tomato

⅓ cup (75 ml) tomatillo salsa

3 Tbsp fresh lime juice

Sea salt and freshly ground black pepper

FOR GARNISH

4 Tbsp (40 g) finely chopped cucumber

4 Tbsp (45 g) finely chopped red onion

½ cup (60 g) halved seedless red grapes

4 tsp chopped fresh cilantro

2 tsp grated lime zest

In a blender, combine the watermelon and tomato. Blend until pulpy, 20–30 seconds. Add the salsa and lime juice and whirl just to combine, 5 seconds. Transfer the soup to a container, cover, and chill thoroughly, at least 4 hours.

To serve, if the soup has separated, shake the container well. Season with salt and pepper. Divide the soup among wide, shallow soup bowls. Add the cucumber, red onion, grapes, cilantro, and lime zest, dividing them evenly among the bowls. Serve right away.

Mushroom Barley Soup with Fresh Thyme

Dried porcini intensify its mushroom flavor and bring the extra savory nuance of umami to this hefty soup. Simmering barley in flavorful broth is an excellent way to get more fiber- and nutrient-rich whole grain into your diet.

4 SERVINGS

½ cup (30 g) dried porcini mushrooms

½ cup (125 ml) dry white wine

1 Tbsp olive oil

2 or 3 large shallots, chopped (about ½ cup/60 g)

2 cloves garlic, minced

8 oz (250 g) fresh cremini mushrooms, brushed clean and chopped

1 tsp minced fresh thyme

Sea salt and freshly ground black pepper

3 cups (700 ml) low-sodium chicken or vegetable broth

¾ cup (150 g) pearl barley

1 Tbsp tomato paste

2 tsp fresh lemon juice

Rinse the porcini well to remove any grit. In a small saucepan over medium-high heat, bring the wine to a simmer. Remove from the heat and add the porcini mushrooms. Let stand for 15 minutes. Drain the porcini over a bowl, reserving the liquid, and chop finely.

In a heavy soup pot over medium-high heat, heat the olive oil. Add the shallots and garlic and cook, stirring often, until the shallots are soft, 2–3 minutes. Add the cremini mushrooms, thyme, ¼ tsp salt, and ¼ tsp pepper and sauté until the cremini release their juices and begin to brown, 4–5 minutes.

Add the porcini-soaking liquid to the pot and bring to a boil, using a wooden spoon to scrape up any browned bits from the pan. Cook for 1 minute.

Add the broth, barley, tomato paste, chopped porcini, and 3 cups (700 ml) water to the pot. Bring to a boil, reduce the heat to medium-low, cover, and simmer gently until the barley is tender, 45–50 minutes.

Transfer about 1 cup (250 ml) of the soup to a blender or food processor and process until smooth. Return the soup to the pot, reheat gently over medium heat just until hot, and stir in the lemon juice. Taste and adjust the seasoning.

Ladle the soup into individual bowls, and serve right away.

Black-Eyed Pea Chowder with Corn & Collard Greens

Collard greens and black-eyed peas, plus the classic Creole trinity of celery, bell pepper, and green onion give this chunky soup Southern flavor. Vegetarians can use Spanish smoked paprika in place of the smoked turkey. Partially cooking the collards before adding them to the chowder reduces overall cooking time.

4 SERVINGS

8 oz (250 g) fresh collard greens, stemmed

2 Tbsp avocado oil or coconut oil

¾ cup (105 g) chopped red onion

½ cup (60 g) sliced celery

½ cup (75 g) chopped green bell pepper

½ cup (45 g) sliced green onions, green and white parts

1 cup (245 g) canned diced tomatoes with jalapeño pepper

2-oz (60-g) piece smoked turkey wing or thigh

3 cups (700 ml) low-sodium vegetable broth

1 Tbsp dried thyme

1 bay leaf

1 can (15 oz/425 g) black-eyed peas, drained and rinsed

1 cup (145 g) fresh or frozen yellow corn kernels

1 Tbsp apple cider vinegar

Sea salt and freshly ground black pepper

In a small Dutch oven or large saucepan, bring 1 cup (250 ml) water to a boil over high heat. Add the collard greens and cook over medium-high heat until they are chewy, 7 minutes. Drain the greens in a colander and set aside until they are cool enough to handle. Chop the greens. Dry the pot.

Meanwhile, in the same pot over medium-high heat, heat the oil until it shimmers. Add the onion, celery, bell pepper, and green onions and cook, stirring occasionally, until the onions have softened, 5 minutes.

Return the chopped collards to the pot. Add the tomatoes, smoked turkey, broth, thyme, and bay leaf. Bring the liquid to a boil over medium-high heat. Reduce the heat, cover, and simmer until the greens are tender, 20 minutes.

Add the black-eyes peas and corn and simmer, covered, until they are heated through. Remove the bay leaf and turkey and discard. Mix in the vinegar and season the chowder with salt and pepper to taste. Divide the chowder among wide, shallow soup bowls. Serve right away.

Smoky Black Bean Soup

Smoked paprika and cumin give Mediterranean flavor to this hearty winter soup. Adding sausage, such as Andouille or kielbasa, brings more intensity and an extra boost of protein. This recipe is easily varied: replace the black beans with white beans to give it even more fiber or swap in chickpeas. Also try parsnips, sweet potato, or shredded cabbage in place of the bell peppers.

4–6 SERVINGS

1 Tbsp olive oil

4 red bell peppers, seeded and diced

3 celery ribs, finely diced

1 yellow onion, finely chopped

1–2 fully cooked smoked turkey, chicken, or pork sausage, chopped

1 tsp ground cumin

1 tsp smoked hot paprika

4 cups (1 l) low-sodium chicken broth

2 cans (15 oz/425 g each) black beans, drained and rinsed

1 can (14.5 oz/411 g) diced tomatoes with juices

Coarse kosher salt and freshly ground black pepper

In a heavy medium pot over medium-high heat, heat the oil. Add the peppers, celery, and onion and sauté until the onion is tender, 5–6 minutes. Add the sausage and sauté until browned, about 2 minutes. Add the cumin and paprika and stir for 1 minute. Add the broth, beans, and tomatoes. Bring the soup to a boil, reduce the heat, and simmer to blend the flavors, at least 20 minutes and up to 45 minutes, thinning with water or more broth as desired.

Season the soup to taste with salt and pepper. Ladle into bowls, and serve right away.

TIP *This soup is fine after 20 minutes of simmering, but it's even better after 45 minutes, or reheated the next day. If the soup gets too thick, thin it to the desired consistency with more broth or water.*

Tofu Kimchi Stew

This Korean soup stars mineral-rich tofu, vitamin-packed cabbage, and fermented kimchi, which aids digestion. Kimchi can be made with or without fish sauce, so if eating vegetarian is important to you, be sure to check the label. You can adjust the heat in this soup by using a mild kimchi and less chile paste. Serve with hot steamed rice.

4 SERVINGS

1 Tbsp avocado oil, coconut oil, or peanut oil

½ yellow onion, thinly sliced

1 cup (100 g) roughly chopped napa cabbage kimchi, plus ½ cup (125 ml) juice from kimchi jar

2 tsp finely chopped garlic

2 tsp peeled and minced fresh ginger

2 cups (500 ml) low-sodium vegetable broth

1 small zucchini, halved lengthwise and sliced into ¼-inch (6-mm) pieces

¼ cup (60 ml) mirin

1–2 Tbsp gochujang or sambal oelek chile paste (optional)

1 tsp sugar

½ lb (250 g) soft tofu

1–2 Tbsp low-sodium soy sauce or tamari

1 tsp dark sesame oil

3 Tbsp thinly sliced green onions, white and pale green parts

In a large saucepan over medium heat, heat the avocado oil. Add the onion and cook until it begins to brown, 4 minutes. Add the chopped kimchi, garlic, and ginger, and cook for 2 minutes.

Add the broth, zucchini, mirin, chile paste (if using), sugar, 2 cups (500 ml) water, and the reserved kimchi juice, and bring to a simmer. Cover and cook until the zucchini is tender, 10 minutes. Break up the tofu into 1-inch (2.5-cm) pieces and gently stir it into the soup. Cook until heated through, 5 minutes. Taste the broth—it should be spicy, sweet, and a little sour from the kimchi.

Adjust the seasoning to taste with soy sauce and additional chile paste, if desired. Stir in the sesame oil, ladle the soup into bowls, sprinkle with the green onions, and serve right away.

TIP *Gochujang is a spicy-sweet red condiment made from red chiles and fermented beans. The thick paste is used extensively in Korean cuisine as a condiment for everything from grilled tofu to soup. You'll usually find it sold in small plastic tubs at Asian markets or online.*

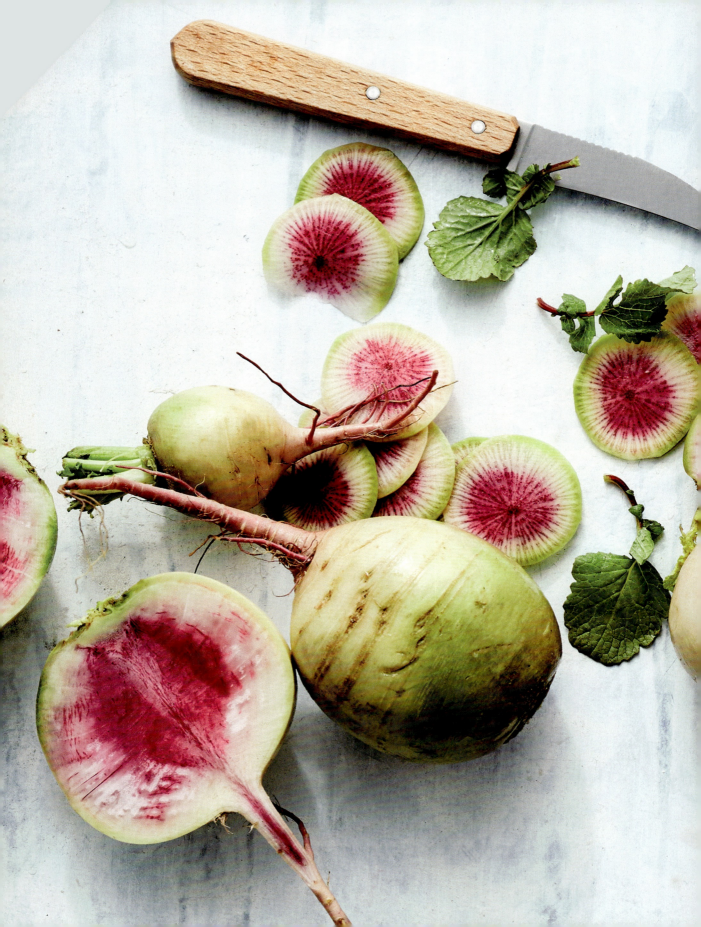

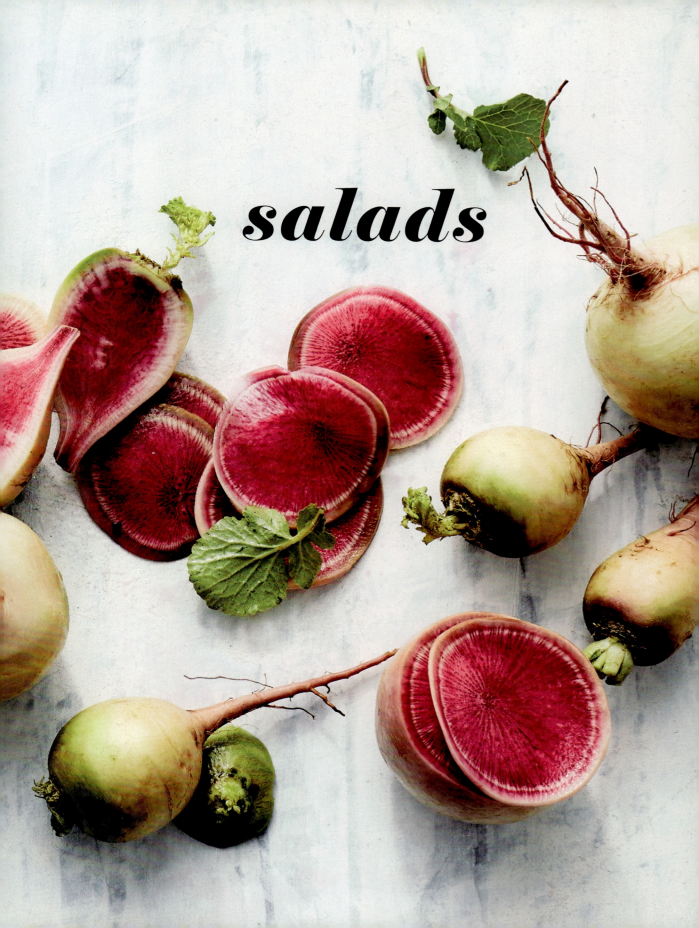

salads

Dungeness Crab & Endive Salad

Along with its sweet and briny taste, crabmeat brings a wealth of minerals, vitamins like B-12, and omega-3s to this dish. It is particularly good when you want less saturated fat than in red meat but still want high quality protein in your diet. It should be noted, however, that crabmeat and other seafood can be high in sodium and should be eaten in moderation if that is a concern.

4-6 SERVINGS

1 lb (500 g) fresh-cooked Dungeness crabmeat, picked over for shell and cartilage fragments

1 watermelon radish, peeled, thinly sliced crosswise, then slices cut in half

½ cucumber, halved lengthwise and thinly sliced crosswise

2 tablespoons minced shallot

Grated zest and juice of 1 lemon

2 tablespoons Champagne vinegar

3 tablespoons extra-virgin olive oil

Kosher salt and freshly ground black pepper

¼ cup (10 g) loosely packed fresh flat-leaf parsley leaves, finely chopped

3 heads Belgian endive

In a large bowl, combine the crabmeat, radish, and cucumber and toss to mix well. In a small bowl, combine the shallot, lemon zest and juice, and vinegar. Whisk in the oil until emulsified, then season to taste with salt and pepper. Drizzle the dressing over the crab mixture and toss gently to coat. Stir in the parsley and season to taste with salt and pepper.

Trim off the base from each endive and separate the leaves. You should have about 15 leaves. Reserve any remainder for another use. Arrange the leaves, hollow side up, and spoon the salad into the bottom 1 inch or so of each leaf. Transfer to a platter and serve.

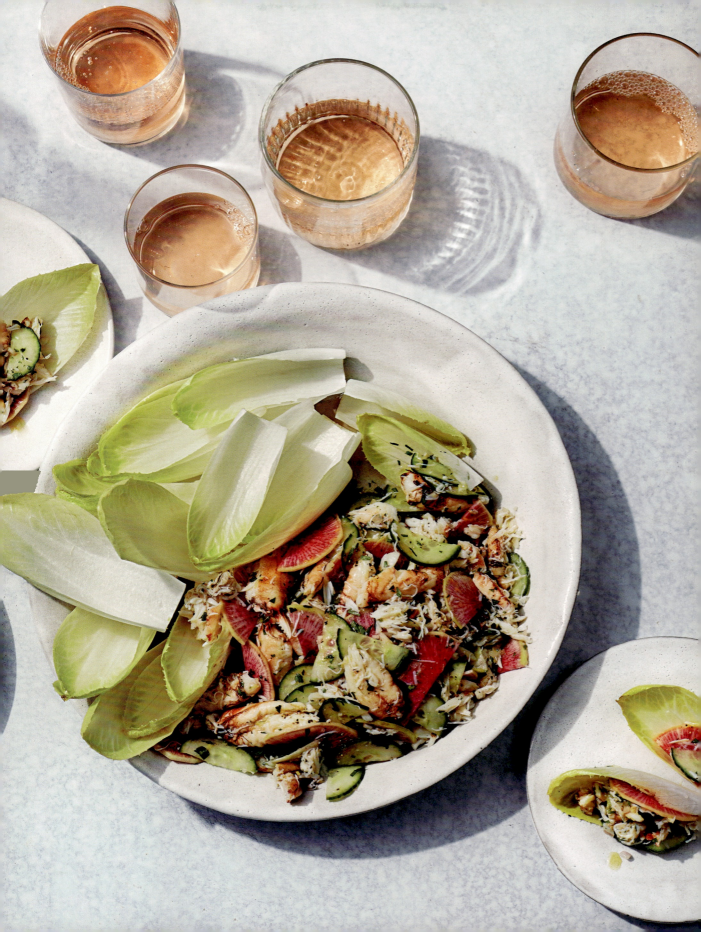

Cucumber Salad with Miso Dressing

This salad is satisfying when you crave something salty and crunchy but healthier than chips. Japanese and Persian cucumbers are slim, with a tender skin and delicate sweetness that is enhanced by the miso dressing. Miso offers immune system boosting benefits from the friendly bacteria found in fermented foods.

4–6 SERVINGS

2 Tbsp white miso

2 Tbsp rice vinegar

2 tsp Asian sesame oil

½ tsp firmly packed light brown sugar

2 lb (1 kg) small Japanese or Persian cucumbers, thinly sliced

2 green onions, white and green parts, thinly sliced

In a bowl, whisk together the miso, vinegar, sesame oil, and brown sugar until well blended. Add the cucumbers and green onion, stir gently to coat with the dressing, and serve.

Indian-Style Chickpea & Tomato Salad

This is a great dish to bring to parties and potlucks. It is an excellent source of micronutrients. Ginger has anti-inflammatory properties and improves digestion, a helpful benefit in this bean salad. If you choose to serve it with romaine lettuce leaves rather than naan, it is a marvelous gluten-free choice.

4 SERVINGS

2 Tbsp olive oil

2 bunches green onions, white and green parts, thinly sliced

1 Tbsp peeled and minced fresh ginger

1 serrano chile, minced with seeds

½ cup (30 g) chopped fresh cilantro

1 ½ tsp ground coriander

2 cans (15.5 oz/439 g each) chickpeas, drained and rinsed

2 Tbsp pomegranate molasses

1 large tomato, seeded and chopped

2 Persian cucumbers, chopped

½ cup (125 g) plain yogurt

¼ tsp ground cumin

Kosher salt and freshly ground black pepper

Romaine heart leaves and/or warmed naan breads, for serving

In a large nonstick frying pan over medium-high heat, heat the oil. Add half of the green onions, the ginger, and the serrano and sauté until tender, about 1 minute. Add ¼ cup (15 g) of the cilantro and the coriander and stir until fragrant, about 30 seconds. Stir in the chickpeas, pomegranate molasses, and ¼ cup (60 ml) water. Simmer until the beans are tender and the liquid is absorbed, about 5 minutes. Let cool slightly.

Meanwhile, in a large bowl, combine the tomato, cucumber, remaining green onions, and remaining ¼ cup (15 g) cilantro. In a small bowl, mix together the yogurt and cumin; season to taste with salt.

Stir the chickpea mixture into the tomato mixture. Season to taste with salt and pepper. Divide the salad among serving plates. Serve with the yogurt sauce, romaine, and/or naan for scooping.

TIP *Keep pomegranate molasses in the cupboard to add a lively sweet-tart taste to salads, sauces, and stewed dishes.*

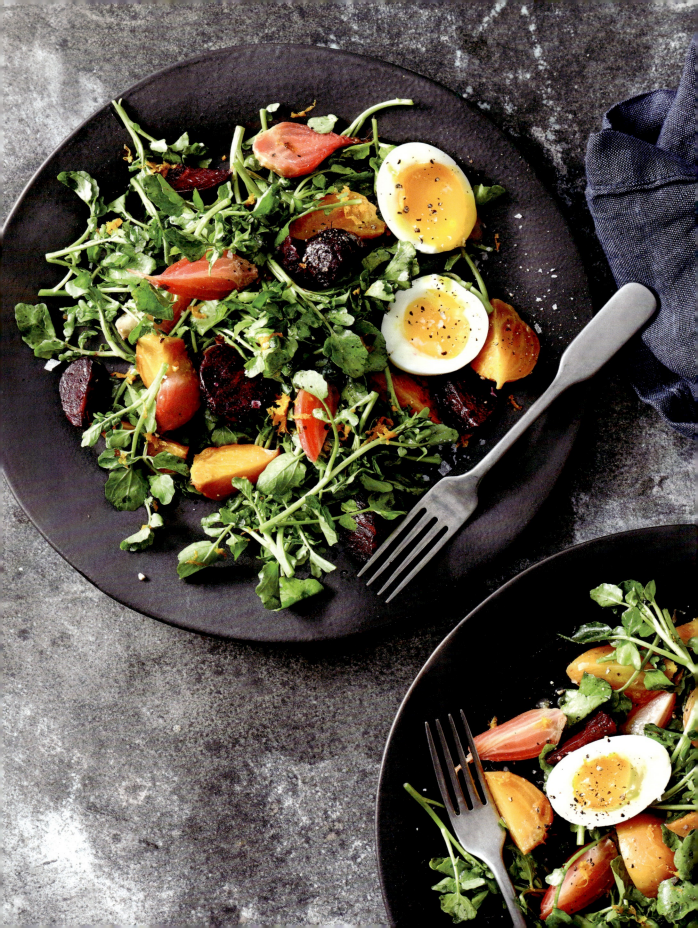

Beet & Watercress Salad with Farm Eggs

Peppery watercress combines well with the sweet, earthy flavor of beets while its mineral profile compliments the array of vitamins in the beets. Use two colors of beets if you like, or striped Chioggia beets if they are available. For the best flavor and rich yolk color, use the freshest possible eggs from a local farm.

4 SERVINGS

1 ½–1 ¾ lb (680–800 g) baby beets

6–8 large organic eggs

Sea salt and freshly ground black pepper

2 Tbsp Champagne vinegar

2 Tbsp fresh orange juice

1 tsp finely grated orange zest

3 Tbsp extra-virgin olive oil

4 cups (4 oz/120 g) watercress, tough stems removed, torn into bite-size pieces

Preheat the oven to 400°F (200°C). Trim the root and stem ends from the beets and wrap them in heavy-duty aluminum foil, making a separate packet for each color, if using. Bake until the beets are pierced easily with a sharp knife, about 45 minutes. Unwrap and let cool. Gently peel the beets with your fingers or a paring knife. Cut into quarters and put in a small bowl.

Place the eggs in a saucepan with enough water to cover by 1 inch (2.5 cm). Bring to a boil over medium-high heat. Remove the pan from the heat, cover, and let stand until done to your liking, about 10 minutes for slightly runny yolks and up to 14 minutes for firm yolks. Drain the eggs, then transfer to a bowl of ice water to cool slightly, 2 minutes or so. Peel the eggs and cut them lengthwise into halves. Sprinkle lightly with salt and pepper.

In a large bowl, stir together the vinegar, orange juice and zest, and ½ tsp salt. Slowly whisk in the olive oil to make a vinaigrette. Pour half of the dressing over the beets and stir to coat. Add the watercress to the bowl with the remaining dressing and toss to coat.

Mound the watercress on individual plates or on a large serving platter and top with the beets. Arrange the egg quarters around the beets and drizzle with any vinaigrette left behind in the watercress bowl. Sprinkle with a few grindings of pepper, and serve right away.

Warm Lentil & Kale Salad

Here, protein- and fiber-rich brown lentils star alongside roasted carrots, sautéed onions, and meaty kale in a salad that shows off bold tastes, contrasting textures, and vibrant colors. A topping of crisped prosciutto adds savory flavor and satisfying fat.

6 SERVINGS

1 Tbsp olive oil

4 carrots, peeled and diced

1 large red onion, thinly sliced

Sea salt and freshly ground black pepper

Leaves from 1 large bunch Tuscan kale, stemmed and thinly sliced

1 cup (200 g) brown lentils, picked over and rinsed

2 sprigs fresh thyme

4 large cloves garlic

4 cups (1 l) low-sodium chicken broth

6 thin slices prosciutto

1 tsp sherry vinegar

In a large saucepan over medium heat, heat the olive oil. Add the carrots and onion, ¼ tsp salt, and several grindings of pepper and sauté until the onion is very soft and lightly caramelized, about 15 minutes. Add the kale leaves to the saucepan and cook, stirring occasionally, until tender, about 6 minutes.

Scrape the contents of the pan into a bowl and set aside. Wipe out the saucepan. In the same saucepan, combine the lentils, thyme, garlic, broth, ½ tsp salt, and ¼ tsp pepper and bring to a boil over high heat.

Reduce the heat to medium and simmer, uncovered, until the lentils are tender but firm to the bite, 15–20 minutes.

Meanwhile, in a frying pan over medium heat, cook the prosciutto until crisp and browned, about 7 minutes. Let cool, then tear into small pieces.

Drain the lentils in the colander, remove and discard the thyme and garlic, and return the lentils to the saucepan. Stir in the kale mixture, vinegar, and ½ tsp salt. Taste and adjust the seasoning. Transfer the lentil mixture to a serving bowl. Top with the prosciutto, and serve right away.

Quinoa with Fresh Herbs & Pomegranate Vinaigrette

The trio of green onion, parsley, and mint, along with summery vegetables, brings verdant color and a bold herbal taste to this refreshing salad. Inspired by traditional Middle Eastern tabbouleh, here protein-rich (and gluten-free!) quinoa stands in for the traditional bulgur. This is a great dish to take to parties.

4 SERVINGS

1 ½ cups (350 g) quinoa

3 cups (700 ml) low-sodium chicken or vegetable broth

Sea salt and freshly ground black pepper

2 large lemons

2 cloves garlic, minced

1 Tbsp pomegranate molasses

1 tsp sugar

½ cup (125 ml) extra-virgin olive oil

2 ripe large tomatoes, seeded and diced

½ large English cucumber, diced

4 green onions, white and pale green parts, thinly sliced

¼ cup (15 g) chopped fresh flat-leaf parsley

¼ cup (15 g) chopped fresh mint

Put the quinoa in a fine-mesh strainer. Rinse thoroughly under cold running water and drain. In a saucepan, bring the broth to a boil over high heat. Add the quinoa and ¼ tsp salt, stir once, and reduce the heat to low. Cover and cook, without stirring, until all the water has been absorbed and the grains are tender, about 15 minutes. Fluff with a fork and transfer to a large bowl.

Finely grate the zest from 1 of the lemons, then halve both lemons and juice the halves to measure 5 Tbsp (75 ml). In a small nonreactive bowl, whisk together the lemon juice and zest, garlic, pomegranate molasses, sugar, tsp salt, and several grindings of pepper until the sugar dissolves. Slowly whisk in the olive oil to make a dressing. Taste and adjust the seasoning. Add about three-fourths of the dressing to the quinoa and stir to mix well.

In a small bowl, toss the tomatoes with ½ tsp salt and let stand until they release their juices, about 5 minutes, then drain in a sieve set over a second bowl.

Place the cucumber along with the green onions in the bowl with the remaining dressing. Toss well, then pour the cucumber mixture over the tomatoes in the sieve to drain. Add the drained tomato-cucumber mixture to the quinoa along with the parsley and mint and stir gently to mix well. Taste, adjust the seasoning, and serve.

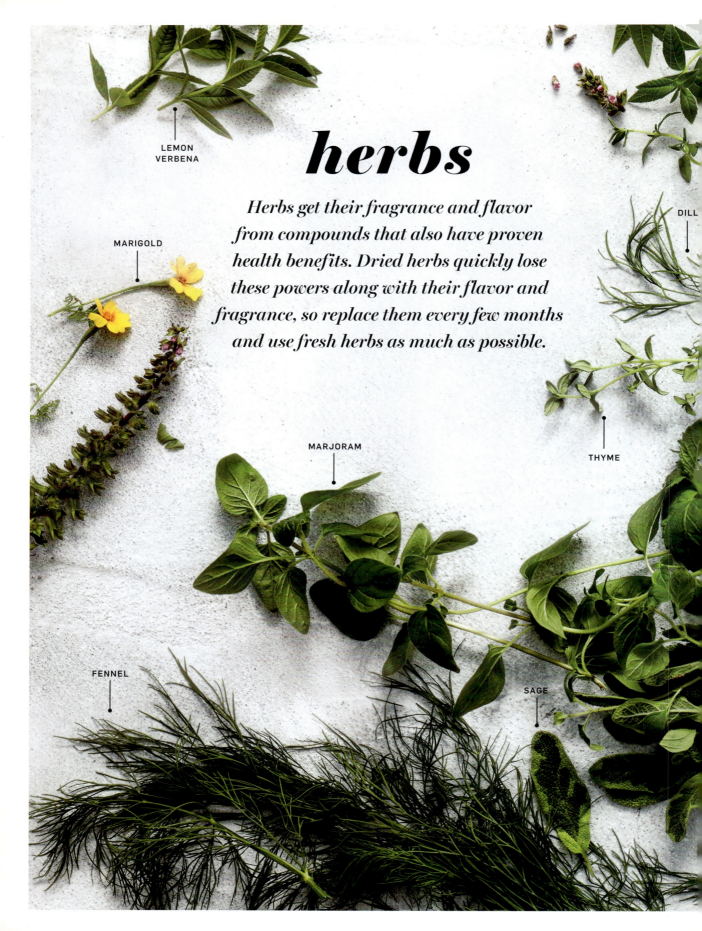

herbs

Herbs get their fragrance and flavor from compounds that also have proven health benefits. Dried herbs quickly lose these powers along with their flavor and fragrance, so replace them every few months and use fresh herbs as much as possible.

LEMON VERBENA

MARIGOLD

DILL

MARJORAM

THYME

FENNEL

SAGE

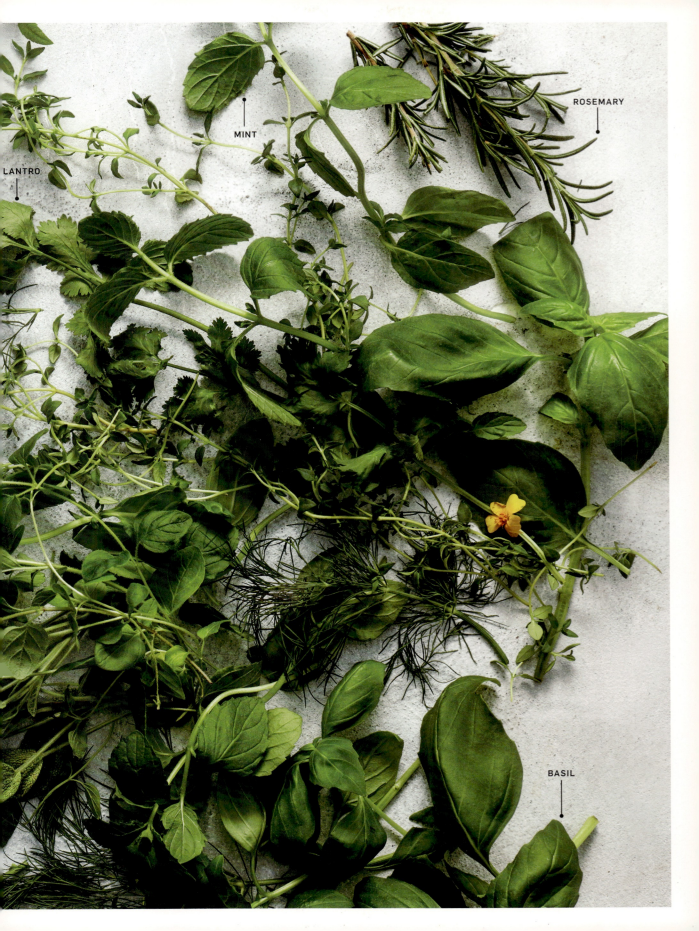

ROSEMARY

MINT

LANTRO

BASIL

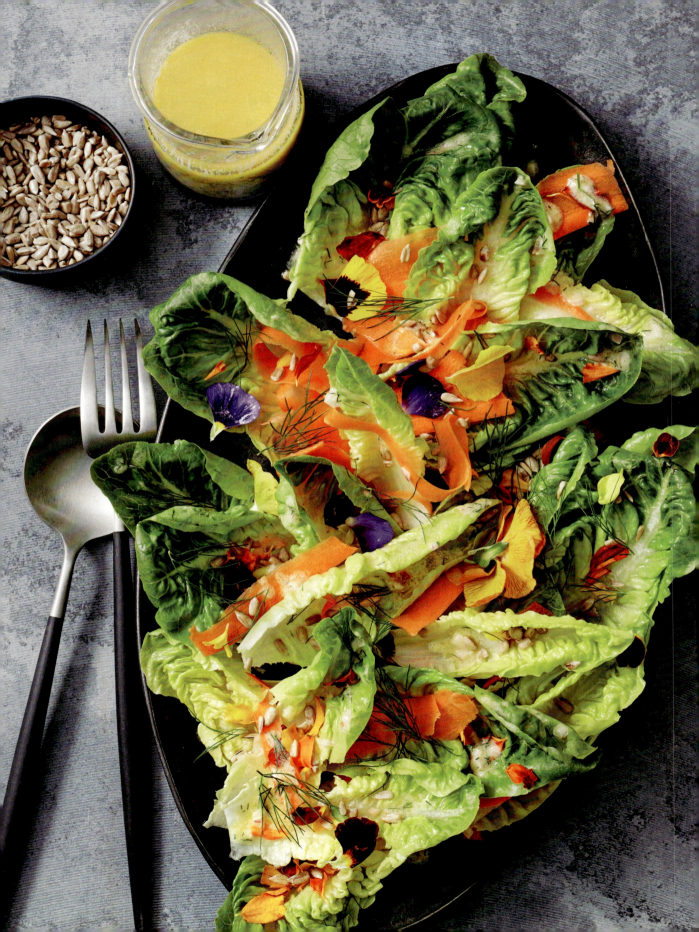

Little Gem Salad with Shaved Carrot, Sunflower Seeds & Dill

Shaved carrots are sprightly, colorful, and mix easily with tender ingredients like the delicate, buttery leaves of Little Gem lettuce. The creamy vinaigrette and crunch of sunflower seeds add pleasing contrast. This dish is high in vitamin A, which helps with immune function, eyesight, and bone health.

6 SERVINGS

FOR THE VINAIGRETTE

2 Tbsp plus 1 tsp Champagne vinegar or white wine vinegar

1 ½ tsp Dijon mustard

1 ½ Tbsp olive-oil mayonnaise

1 shallot, minced

Sea salt and freshly ground black pepper

6 Tbsp (90 ml) extra-virgin olive oil

2 ½ Tbsp finely chopped fresh dill

4 heads Little Gem lettuce (about 12 oz/350 g total weight), leaves separated

1 large carrot, peeled and shaved paper-thin

⅔ cup (80 g) sunflower seeds

Handful of nasturtium leaves and/or blossoms, for garnish (optional)

To make the vinaigrette, in a large salad bowl, stir together the vinegar, mustard, mayonnaise, shallot, ¾ tsp salt, and pepper to taste until well combined. Slowly whisk in the olive oil to make a vinaigrette. Stir in the dill.

Add the lettuce, carrot, and half of the sunflower seeds to the salad bowl and toss to combine. Scatter with the remaining sunflower seeds and some nasturtium leaves and/or blossoms, if using, and serve.

White Bean, Tuna & Fennel Salad

Tuna is a powerhouse ingredient containing all nine essential amino acids that make up a complete protein. Omega-3 fatty acids, vitamins, and minerals add even more to it's robust nutrition. Combining the fish with white beans make this a substantial salad that will keep you full and satisfied for hours.

4 SERVINGS

2 fennel bulbs, trimmed

2 cans (15 oz/425 g each) cannellini beans, rinsed and drained

2 cans (5 oz/150 g each) albacore tuna in olive oil, drained and broken into large pieces

½ cup (60 g) finely chopped red onion

½ cup (75 g) pitted Kalamata olives, quartered lengthwise

¼ cup (15 g) chopped fresh mint

2 tsp Dijon mustard

2 Tbsp fresh lemon juice

⅓ cup (75 ml) extra-virgin olive oil

Kosher salt and freshly ground black pepper

1 head butter lettuce or romaine lettuce

DF SF

Cut the fennel bulbs lengthwise into quarters, cut out the core if it seems tough, and then slice crosswise. In a large bowl, combine the fennel, beans, tuna, onion, olives, and mint.

In a small bowl, stir together the mustard and lemon juice. Slowly whisk in the olive oil to make a dressing and season with a generous amount of pepper. Pour over the salad and gently toss. Season to taste with salt and additional pepper.

Line serving plates with lettuce leaves, or arrange them on a platter. Mound the salad on top of the lettuce, and serve.

TIP *Look for line-caught canned albacore tuna for a sustainable choice. Canned wild Alaskan salmon is a good alternative. Try leftovers mounded on rice crackers as a snack the next day.*

Farro, Corn & Runner Bean Salad

Make this dish early on a summer's day to enjoy for dinner or at an impromptu potluck. Farro, an often-overlooked ancient form of wheat, provides protein and fiber. Use brown ride for a gluten-free version. For a beautiful presentation, line the edge of a platter with sliced tomatoes and spoon the salad in the center.

4 SERVINGS

Kosher salt and freshly ground black pepper

½ cup (90 g) farro

¾ lb (350 g) runner beans or green beans, trimmed and cut into 1 ½-inch (4-cm) lengths

2 cups (360 g) yellow corn kernels (from about 2 ears)

3 green onions, white and pale green parts, thinly sliced

2 Tbsp extra-virgin olive oil

1 Tbsp minced fresh marjoram leaves, plus 2 tsp whole leaves

2 Tbsp white wine vinegar

1 clove garlic, pressed

2 tsp Dijon mustard

1 cup (4 oz/120 g) crumbled goat cheese

Bring a large saucepan three-fourths full of salted water to a boil. Add the farro and boil until just tender, 25–30 minutes. Drain and let cool.

Refill the saucepan three-fourths full with salted water and bring to a boil. Add the beans and cook until tender-crisp, about 4 minutes. Drain and plunge into cold water to cool. Drain again.

In a large serving bowl, combine the farro, green beans, corn, and green onions. In a small bowl, muddle together the olive oil, minced marjoram, and ¼ tsp salt. Whisk in the vinegar, garlic, and mustard. Pour the dressing over the salad and toss well. Season with salt and pepper, then sprinkle with the goat cheese and marjoram leaves and serve.

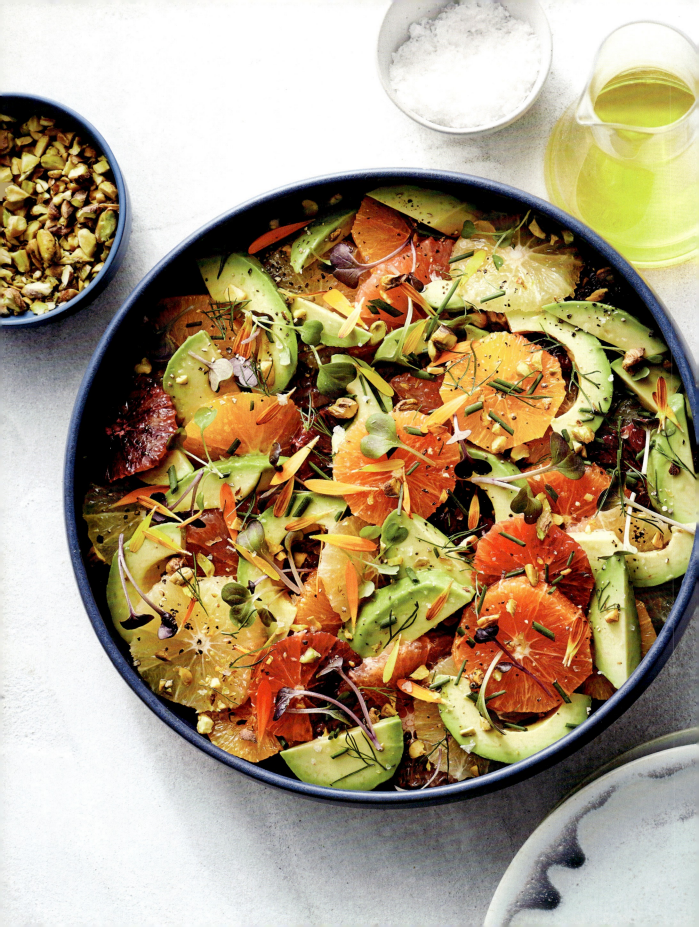

Avocado Citrus Salad

This cheerful salad is the perfect starter or light lunch to brighten both your table and your mood. Think of it especially when you are doing a detox. Its citrus is packed with minerals and vitamins, including a healthy dose of C for an immune boost, plus other antioxidants that help reduce inflammation. Avocado and nuts bring healthy fats to keep you satisfied.

6 SERVINGS

8 citrus fruits, in assorted types and colors as desired (try Cara Cara, blood, and navel oranges and pink and red grapefruits)

3 avocados, pitted, peeled, and sliced

¼ cup (30 g) pistachios, toasted and roughly chopped

Good-quality extra-virgin olive oil, for drizzling

Flaky sea salt and freshly ground black pepper

Assorted fresh herbs (such as fennel fronds and micro arugula) and edible flowers, for garnish

VG · V · GF · DF · SF

To peel each citrus, using a sharp knife, cut off a thin slice from the top and bottom of the fruit to expose the flesh. Stand the citrus, cut side down, on a work surface. Using a gentle sawing motion and following the contour of the fruit, cut downward to remove all the peel and white pith, working your way around the fruit. Slice each fruit crosswise into rounds about ¼ inch (6 mm) thick.

Arrange the citrus and avocado slices on a serving plate. Sprinkle with the pistachios and top with a generous drizzle of your finest oil. Season with salt and pepper, garnish with herbs and flowers, and serve.

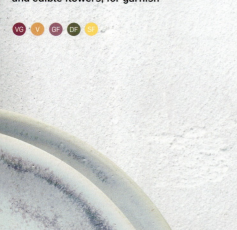
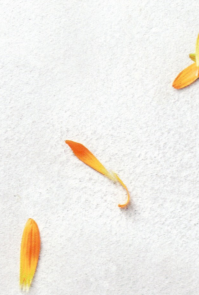
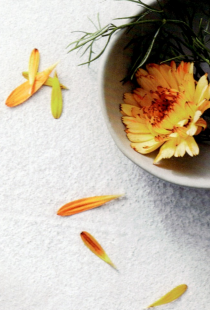

Chopped Salad of Peppers, Tomatoes & Olives

A beautiful presentation and easy assembly make this colorful salad perfect for entertaining. Nutritionally, it fits many dietary preferences, especially if you serve the Manchego cheese on the side and skip the anchovies in the Green Goddess Dressing.

6 SERVINGS

Avocado Green Goddess Dressing (page 186)

1 small yellow bell pepper, seeded and chopped

1 small orange bell pepper, seeded and chopped

2 cups (375 g) cherry or grape tomatoes, halved

4 ribs celery, thinly sliced

¾ cup (105 g) pitted large green olives, quartered

¼ cup (45 g) finely chopped red onion

1 Tbsp chopped fresh flat-leaf parsley

1 tsp chopped fresh thyme

8 oz (250 g) Manchego cheese, cut into ¼-inch (6-mm) cubes (optional)

Sea salt and freshly ground black pepper

Into a large salad bowl, spoon ½ cup (125 ml) dressing. Add the bell peppers, tomatoes, celery, olives, onion, parsley, thyme, and cheese, if using, to the dressing in the bowl. Toss until all the ingredients are coated with the dressing, adding more dressing as desired. Season with salt and pepper to taste. Serve right away.

Watermelon Radish Salad with Avocado Vinaigrette

Radishes come in a wide range of sizes, shapes, and colors. Besides the familiar round red ones, varieties include thin white icicle radishes; Easter egg radishes in purple, white, lavender, or pink; French breakfast radishes that are elongated, two-tone red and white; pungent black radishes; and watermelon radishes with their combination of pale green skin and pinkish red flesh. All radishes get their spicy bite from sulfur-related substances that help protect against cancer.

4 SERVINGS

1 shallot, finely diced

1 ½ Tbsp fresh lemon juice, plus extra if needed

1 ½ Tbsp white wine vinegar

Sea salt

¼ cup (60 ml) extra-virgin olive oil

1 avocado, halved, pitted, and diced

2 heads romaine lettuce, dark outer leaves cut into ½-inch (12-mm) pieces

1 watermelon radish, thinly sliced

¼ cup (15 g) chopped fresh cilantro

In a large salad bowl, stir together the shallot, the 1½ Tbsp lemon juice, vinegar, and a pinch of salt. Slowly whisk in the olive oil to make a vinaigrette. Gently stir in the avocado and let stand for 10 minutes, stirring occasionally.

Add the romaine, radish, and cilantro to the salad bowl. Toss gently with the vinaigrette and avocado and season to taste with additional salt and lemon juice. Serve right away.

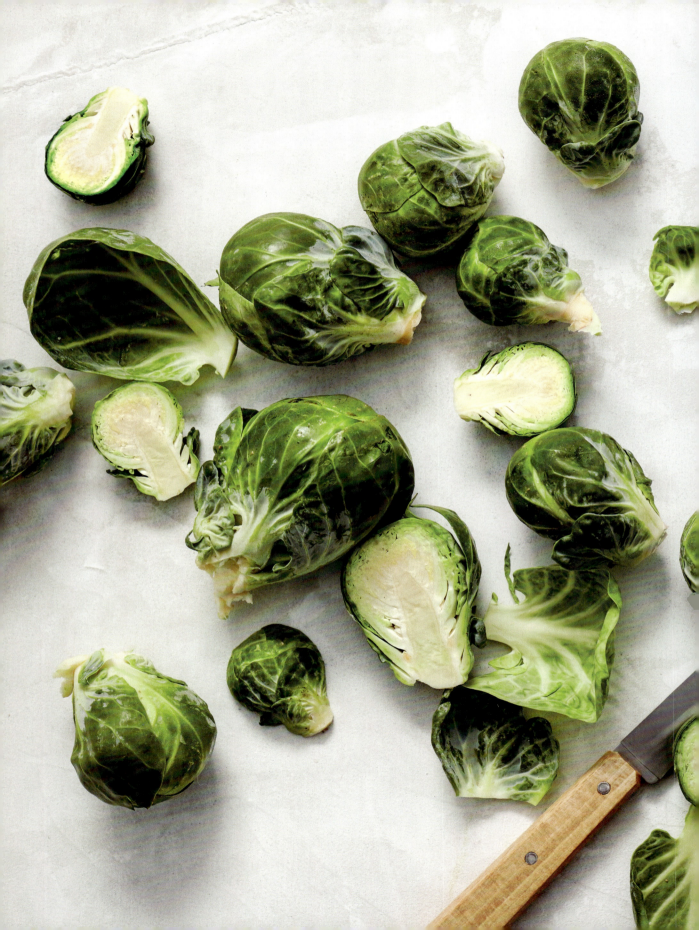

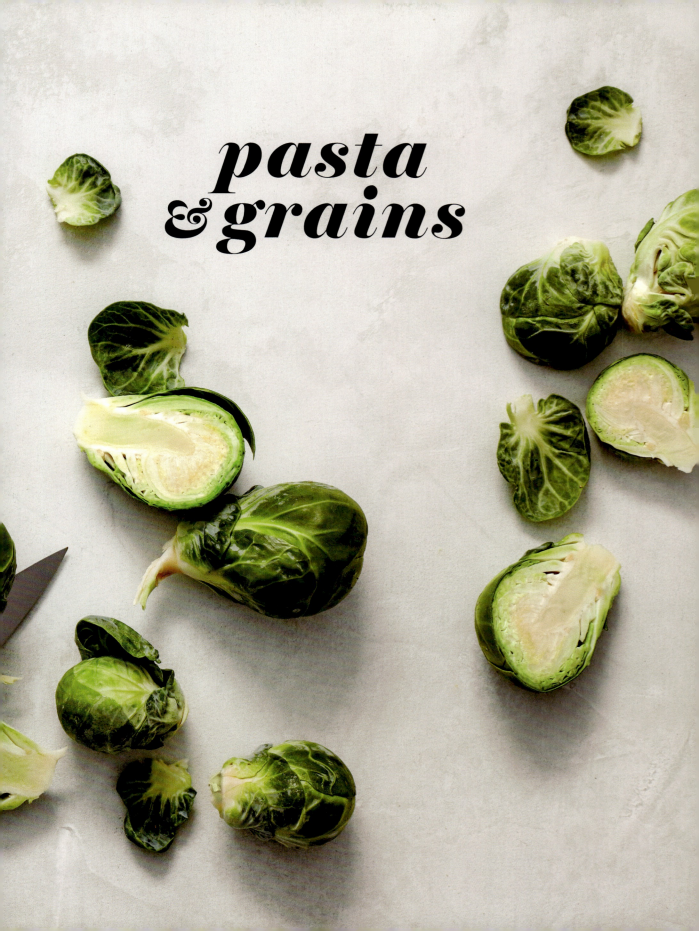

pasta
& grains

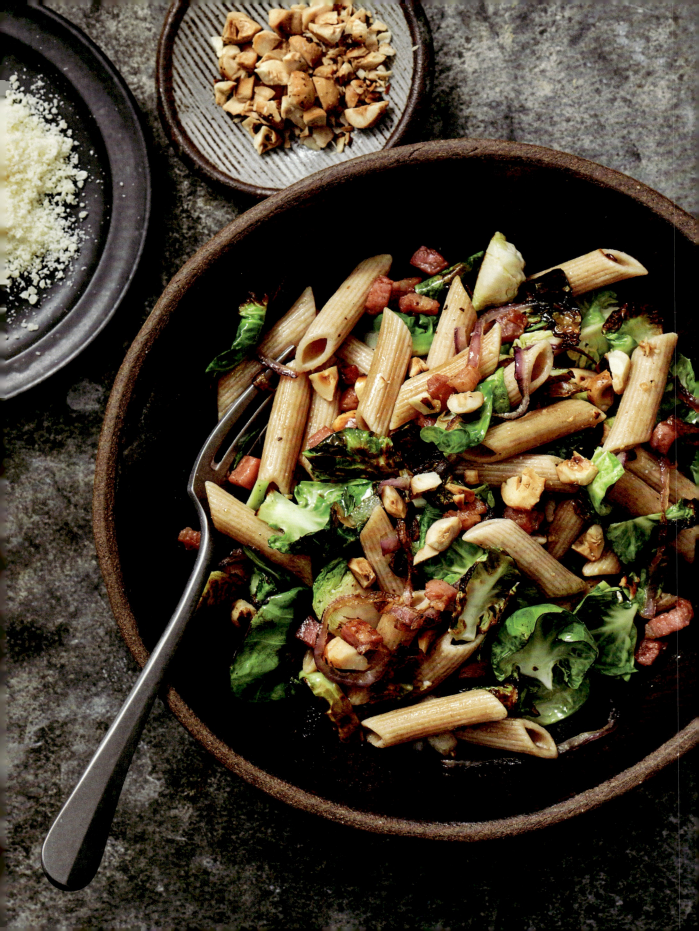

Pasta with Brussels Sprout Leaves, Hazelnuts & Brown Butter

Brussels sprouts are a proud member of the super-healthful crucifer family. We tend to think of roasting them whole or halved but pulling apart the individual leaves is another delicious option. This task is time consuming, so recruit a friend to help and pour some wine to make the job go more quickly. The results are worth it!

4 SERVINGS

6 Tbsp (90 g) unsalted butter

½ cup (75 g) hazelnuts, coarsely chopped

14 oz (400 g) Brussels sprouts

1 ½ Tbsp olive-oil mayonnaise mixed with 2 Tbsp olive oil

Kosher salt and freshly ground black pepper

2 thick slices pancetta (about 3 oz/90 g total weight), finely chopped

1 red onion, very thinly sliced

¾ lb (350 g) whole-grain penne pasta

Preheat the broiler. In a small saucepan, combine the butter and hazelnuts. Place over medium-high heat and melt the butter, swirling until foamy and nut brown. Remove from the heat and set aside.

Quarter the Brussels sprouts through the core. Trim away the triangular core from each quarter, then break or pull apart into leaves. On a large rimmed baking sheet, toss together the Brussels sprout leaves and mayonnaise–olive oil mixture until evenly coated. Spread in an even layer and season generously with salt and pepper. Broil until nicely charred in places but not blackened, 3–5 minutes, tossing once partway through the cooking. Set aside.

In a large frying pan over medium-low heat, heat 1 Tbsp olive oil. Add the pancetta and onion and cook, stirring occasionally, until the onion is softened, about 15 minutes. Remove from the heat.

Meanwhile, bring a large pot of salted water to a boil. Add the pasta and stir well. Cook, stirring occasionally, until al dente, according to the package directions. Drain well, reserving ¼ cup (60 ml) of the cooking water.

Add the cooking water to the pan with the onion and place back over medium-low heat. Fold in the pasta and half of the Brussels sprout leaves until blended and season generously with salt and pepper. Heat until warmed through, about 1 minute, then transfer to a platter. Place the hazelnut butter over medium heat and quickly return to a sizzle. Spoon the bubbling butter and hazelnuts over the pasta. Scatter the remaining sprout leaves on top, and serve.

Penne with Walnut Pesto & Peas

Walnuts contain twice as many immune-boosting antioxidants than any other nut. Replace the usual pine nuts in pesto with walnuts to take full advantage of their benefits in a delicious way! This all-purpose sauce is also good over chicken or tossed with broccoli. Experiment with the many different types and shapes of whole-grain pastas available to discover your favorite.

4 SERVINGS

2 cups (60 g) packed fresh basil leaves

2 shallots or 1 clove garlic, coarsely chopped

¼ cup (30 g) walnuts

2 tsp finely grated lemon zest

Kosher salt and freshly ground black pepper

¼ cup (60 ml) extra-virgin olive oil

¼ cup (1 oz/30 g) freshly grated pecorino romano cheese, plus more as needed

¾ lb (350 g) whole-grain penne pasta

10 oz (280 g) sugar snap peas, strings removed

10 oz (280 g) shelled English peas or 1 package (10 oz/280 g) frozen peas

In a food processor, combine the basil, shallots, walnuts, lemon zest, and ½ tsp salt. Process until finely ground. With the machine running, gradually add the olive oil. Mix in the ¼ cup (30 g) cheese. Season to taste with salt and a generous amount of pepper.

Bring a large pot of salted water to a boil. Add the pasta and stir well. Cook, stirring occasionally, for about 4 minutes less than the cooking time indicated on the package. Add the sugar snaps and English peas and cook until the pasta is al dente, stirring occasionally, about 4 minutes longer.

When the pasta is ready, reserve ¾ cup (180 ml) of the cooking water and drain the pasta and peas. Put the pesto in a large bowl. Whisk in enough of the reserved cooking water to thin it to a sauce. Add the pasta and vegetables and toss to coat. Thin with more cooking liquid as needed and season with salt. Serve right away, passing additional cheese at the table.

Whole-Wheat Spaghetti with Mushroom Bolognese Sauce

This vegetarian take on Bologna's renowned meat sauce has the same rich layering of flavors. Selenium in mushrooms supports your immune system. Red wine brings healthful antioxidants. For a cholesterol-free, vegan option, replace the cream with coconut nondairy creamer. This sauce merits using the best-quality San Marzano tomatoes. Farro or spelt pasta works well here.

6 SERVINGS

¾ cup (105 g) coarsely chopped red onion

¾ cup (90 g) coarsely chopped carrot

¾ cup (90 g) coarsely chopped celery

2 Tbsp olive oil

3 cloves garlic, chopped

1 lb (500 g) cremini mushrooms, stemmed and quartered

1 Tbsp dried thyme

1 tsp freshly grated nutmeg

½ cup (120 ml) dry red wine

¼ cup (2 ½ oz/70 g) tomato paste

1 can (28 oz/800 g) peeled Roma (plum) tomatoes, juices reserved

3 Tbsp cream

Sea salt and freshly ground black pepper

1 lb (500 g) whole-wheat spaghetti

Chopped fresh flat-leaf parsley, for garnish (optional)

In a food processor, combine the onion, carrot, and celery and pulse until they are very finely chopped and moist.

In a medium-sized, deep frying pan over medium-high heat, heat the olive oil. When the oil shimmers, add the chopped vegetables. Cook, stirring often, for 5 minutes. Add the garlic and cook, stirring, until the vegetables are very soft, about 5 minutes more. Take care not to let them brown.

Add the mushrooms and cook, stirring occasionally, until they look wet, 5 minutes. Mix in the thyme and nutmeg. Continue cooking until the mushrooms are almost dry, 4 minutes. Pour in the wine and cook until it is almost evaporated, 8 minutes. Mix in the tomato paste.

One at a time, add the tomatoes, cutting each into 8 pieces with a pair of kitchen shears. Add 1 cup (250 ml) of their liquid. Simmer the sauce until it looks meaty, with a sheen on the surface, 10 minutes. Mix in the cream and simmer the sauce for 5 minutes. Season with salt and pepper to taste.

While the sauce is simmering, bring a large pot of salted water to a boil. When the sauce is nearly done, add the pasta and stir well. Cook according to package directions. Drain and divide it among pasta bowls. Ladle the sauce over the pasta. Garnish with the parsley, if desired. Serve at once.

Quinoa & Avocado Bowl with Tahini Dressing

Our love affair with avocado is easy to understand: besides being lusciously creamy, this super fruit is loaded with fiber, antioxidants, and 20 vitamins and minerals. It is high in fat, but its monounsaturated fats help lower bad cholesterol, which helps reduce the risk of heart disease and stroke.

4 SERVINGS

2 fennel bulbs, trimmed and cut lengthwise into wedges ¾ inch (2 cm) thick

1 Tbsp olive oil

Kosher salt

1 cup (180 g) quinoa, rinsed and drained

FOR THE TAHINI DRESSING

½ cup (120 g) tahini

1 clove garlic, grated

2 Tbsp fresh lemon juice

1 tsp grated lemon zest

6 Tbsp (90 ml) warm water

1 tsp honey

2 avocados, halved, pitted, and sliced

2 Persian cucumbers, sliced

1 cup (225 g) cherry tomatoes, halved

1 bunch rainbow radishes, thinly sliced

½ cup (2 oz/60 g) crumbled feta cheese

Fresh mint leaves, for garnish

Black sesame seeds, for garnish

Preheat the oven to 425°F (220°C). Pile the fennel wedges on a baking sheet, drizzle with the oil, sprinkle with a pinch of salt, and toss to coat. Spread the wedges in a single layer and roast until they begin to brown, soften, and caramelize, about 15 minutes.

Meanwhile, in a saucepan over high heat, combine the quinoa, 2 cups (500 ml) water, and a generous pinch of salt and bring to a boil over high heat. Reduce the heat to low, cover, and cook until the quinoa is tender, about 15 minutes. Remove from the heat and let stand for 5 minutes.

To make the tahini dressing, in a bowl, whisk together the tahini, garlic, lemon juice and zest, water, and honey, mixing well. Season to taste with salt.

Divide the quinoa among serving bowls. Top with the fennel, avocado, cucumber, tomatoes, radishes, and feta, arranging them attractively. Drizzle with the tahini dressing, garnish with mint and sesame seeds, and serve warm or at room temperature.

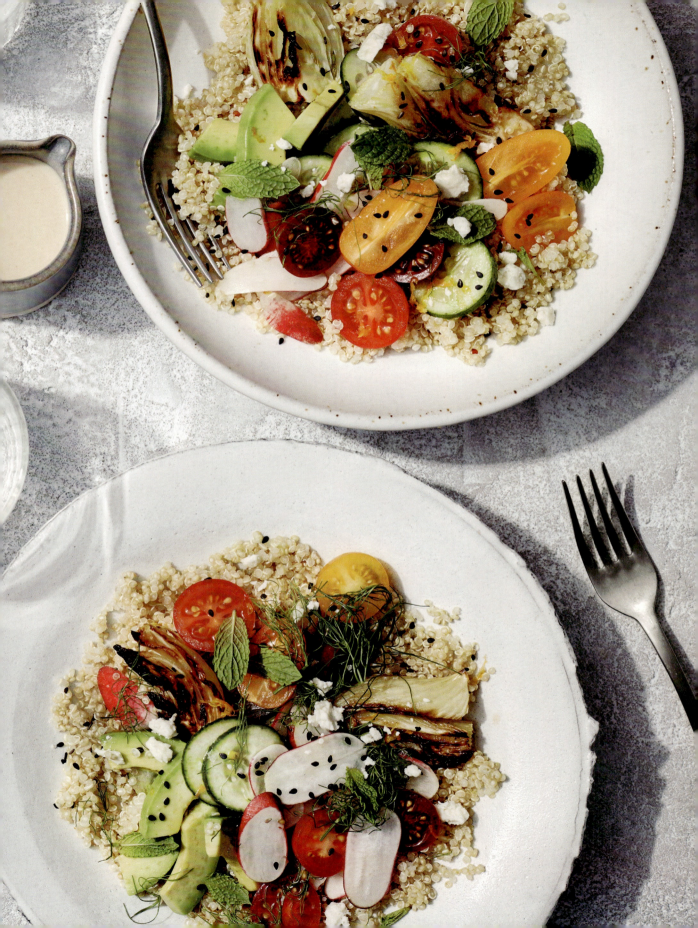

Quinoa Spaghetti with Broccoli Rabe, Feta & Mint

Broccoli rabe looks like a leggy cousin of broccoli but it's actually botanically closer to turnips. Mellow its somewhat bitter, assertive bite by blanching it, then pair broccoli rabe with nutty quinoa pasta for a hearty midweek meal.

4 SERVINGS

1 lb (500 g) broccoli rabe

¾ lb (350 g) quinoa or other whole-grain spaghetti

¼ cup (60 ml) olive oil

6 large cloves garlic, thinly sliced

Pinch of red chile flakes

Sea salt and freshly ground black pepper

1 cup (4 oz/120 g) crumbled feta cheese

1 cup (120 g) walnuts, toasted and roughly chopped

⅓ cup (13 g) chopped fresh mint leaves

Cut the broccoli rabe stems into bite-sized lengths and set aside. Roughly chop the leaves and florets, keeping them separate from the stems. Bring a large pot of salted water to a boil. Add the stems to the water and boil for 1 minute. Add the leaves and florets to the water and boil until wilted and just tender, about 3 minutes longer. Using a fine-mesh sieve or slotted spoon, quickly remove the broccoli rabe from the cooking water and drain in a colander, shaking off any excess water still clinging to the leaves.

Return the cooking water to a boil, add the pasta, and cook until al dente, according to package directions.

While the pasta is cooking, in a large frying pan over medium heat, heat the oil. Add the garlic and sauté until aromatic, 1 minute. Add the reserved broccoli rabe and red chile flakes, and sauté for 1 minute. Season with salt and pepper, then reduce the heat to low to keep warm.

When the pasta is ready, reserve ¾ cup (180 ml) of the cooking water and drain the pasta. Add the pasta to the broccoli rabe in the frying pan along with the cheese, walnuts, and mint. Toss to combine, adding as much of the reserved cooking water as needed to moisten the pasta. Serve right away.

TIP *Look for broccoli rabe that has fresh—not split—stems, lots of green leaves, and deep green florets. Avoid bunches that have yellowing flowers or dry-looking stem ends. For this recipe, the softer and creamier the feta, the better. Choose a mild French feta if available.*

Soba Noodles with Asparagus, Shiitake Mushrooms & Wakame

This Japanese-inspired dish is perfect to highlight asparagus at its peak in late spring. Wakame, a deep-green sea vegetable, adds briny counterpoint to the asparagus. Soba noodles add protein to this nutrient-rich entrée. Unless labeled 100 percent buckwheat, soba noodles also contain wheat flour.

4 SERVINGS

2 Tbsp dried wakame or mixed sea vegetables

2 Tbsp low-sodium soy sauce

2 Tbsp rice vinegar

1 tsp sugar

2 tsp toasted sesame oil

¾ lb (350 g) soba noodles

2 Tbsp avocado oil, coconut oil, or peanut oil

2 tsp peeled and grated fresh ginger

2 tsp finely chopped garlic

¾ lb (350 g) thin asparagus, trimmed and cut into 2-inch (5-cm) lengths

1 cup (90 g) shiitake mushrooms, stems discarded and caps sliced

In a bowl, combine the wakame with 1 cup (250 ml) cold water. Set aside to soften for 15 minutes. Drain, squeeze out the excess water, and set aside.

In a small bowl, whisk together the soy sauce, vinegar, sugar, and sesame oil until the sugar dissolves; set aside.

Bring a pot of water to a boil. Add the soba noodles and cook until just tender, about 4 minutes. Drain and rinse with cool water to stop them from overcooking; set aside.

In a wok or large nonstick frying pan over medium-high heat, heat the avocado oil. Add the ginger and garlic and stir-fry until aromatic, 20 seconds. Add the asparagus and mushrooms and stir-fry for 1 minute. Add 2 Tbsp water, cover, and cook until the asparagus is tender-crisp and bright green, about 2 minutes, depending on their thickness.

Uncover, remove the pan from heat, and add the noodles and the soy sauce mixture, tossing to coat. Divide the noodle-vegetable mixture among shallow bowls. Top the noodles with the wakame and serve warm or at room temperature.

> **TIP** *Soba noodles come in a variety of types, from 100 percent buckwheat to a mix of mostly white flour with some buckwheat added for color. The more buckwheat in the noodles, the more intense their flavor—and the higher their price tag. If you're crunched for time, you can substitute fresh yakisoba (available in the produce department of well-stocked supermarkets) for the soba: Just drop the precooked noodles directly into the wok to reheat them. Look for dried wakame or mixed sea vegetable packets at natural foods markets, Asian stores, or online—they're well worth the hunt!*

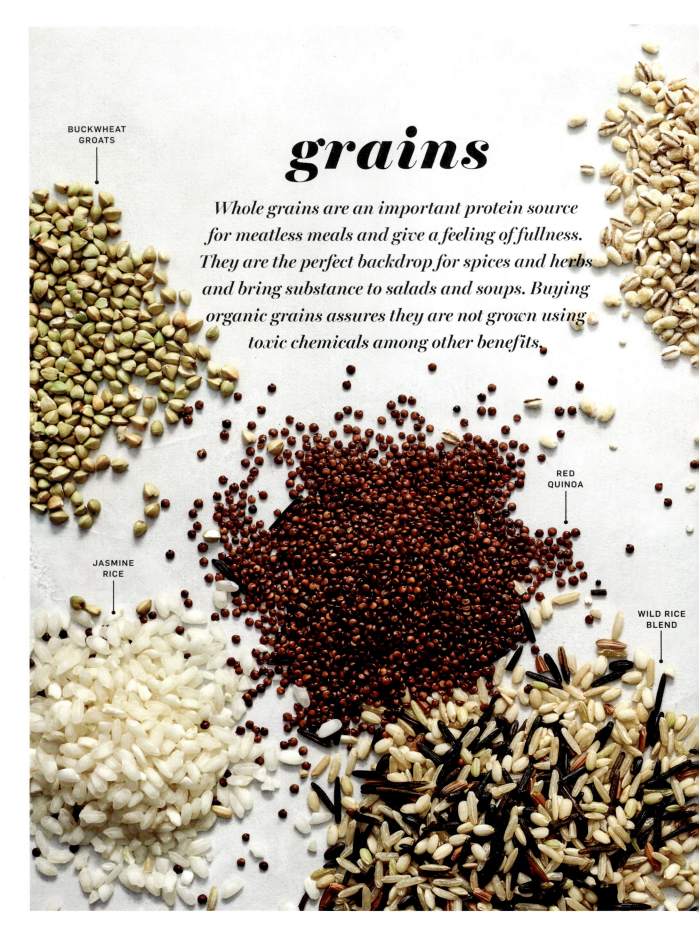

BUCKWHEAT
GROATS

grains

Whole grains are an important protein source for meatless meals and give a feeling of fullness. They are the perfect backdrop for spices and herbs and bring substance to salads and soups. Buying organic grains assures they are not grown using toxic chemicals among other benefits.

RED
QUINOA

JASMINE
RICE

WILD RICE
BLEND

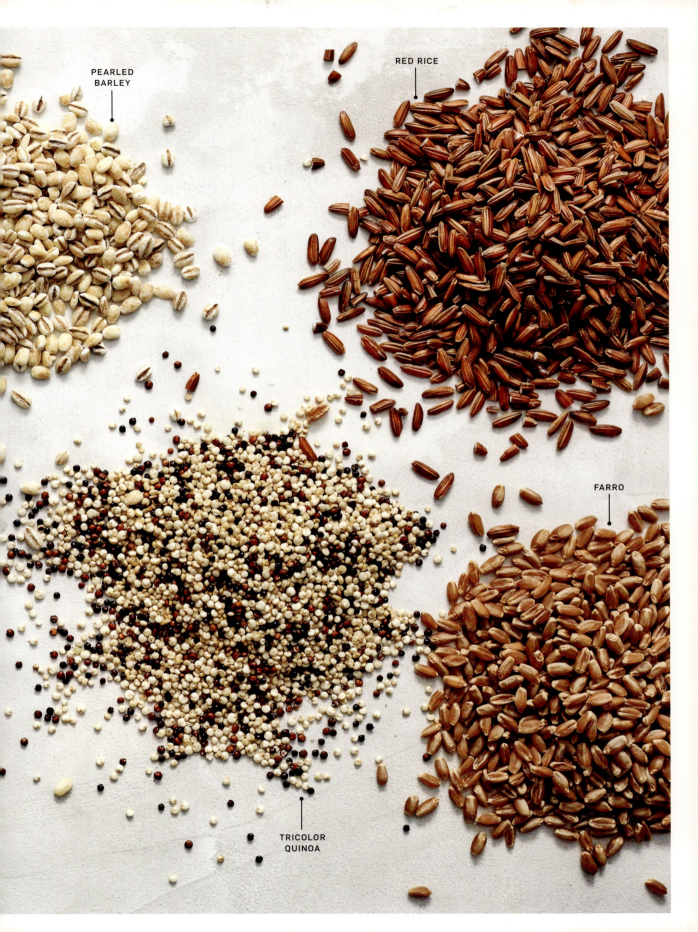

PEARLED
BARLEY

RED RICE

FARRO

TRICOLOR
QUINOA

Wild Rice & Mushroom Pilaf

Cooks divide mushrooms into two categories: cultivated, including white button mushrooms, cremini, and meaty portobello; and "wild" (though generally cultivated nowadays), like versatile shiitake, Italian porcini, delicate oyster mushrooms, and apricot-scented chanterelles. All are wonderful sources of micronutrients, including selenium that helps repair DNA. Use any types you like here.

6 SERVINGS

1 Tbsp unsalted butter or olive oil

1 small leek, white part only, chopped

1 lb (500 g) mixed fresh mushrooms such as white button, shiitake, and chanterelle, brushed clean, tough stems trimmed or discarded

1 cup (160 g) wild rice, rinsed and drained

¼ cup (15 g) chopped fresh flat-leaf parsley

Kosher salt and freshly ground black pepper

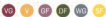

In a large saucepan over medium heat, melt the butter or heat the oil. Add the leek and the mushrooms and sauté until the leeks are soft and translucent and the mushrooms begin to brown, about 8 minutes.

Add the wild rice and parsley, season with salt and pepper, and add water to cover by 1 inch (2.5 cm). Bring to a boil, reduce the heat to low, cover, and cook until the rice is tender, about 45 minutes. (The cooking time will vary with different batches of rice.) The wild rice is ready when the grains puff up and the inner, lighter part is visible. Drain off any excess water.

Transfer to a serving dish and serve right away.

Barley with Kale & Lemon

Barley is often an overlooked grain that, like oatmeal, is rich in both soluble and insoluble fiber. Combining it with kale creates a dish that satisfies as a meatless main course and is also perfect when accompanied by sausages or roasted chicken.

4 SERVINGS

Kosher salt

½ cup (100 g) pearl barley

1 bunch lacinato kale
(about 1 lb/500 g)

2 Tbsp olive oil

1 small yellow onion, finely
chopped

4 cloves garlic, chopped

¼ tsp red chile flakes

½ tsp grated lemon zest

1–2 Tbsp fresh lemon juice

Bring a large saucepan half full of salted water to a boil over high heat. Add the barley and cook until tender, about 45 minutes. Drain and set aside.

Meanwhile, cut the tough stems from the kale leaves. Stack the leaves, roll them up lengthwise, and cut crosswise into thin strips. Discard the stems.

In a large, heavy frying over medium-high heat, heat the olive oil. Add the onion and sauté until golden brown, about 6 minutes. Add the garlic and sauté until fragrant, about 1 minute. Reduce the heat to medium, add the kale, and sprinkle with the red chile flakes. Sauté until the kale is tender and wilted, about 7 minutes. Stir in the lemon zest and season with salt, then add the lemon juice to taste.

Transfer to a serving dish and serve.

Coconut Rice with Black Beans & Collard Greens

Black beans are higher in fiber and protein than the small red ones Jamaican cooks use. Starting the greens in a small amount of water produces enough vitamin-rich pot liquor to finish cooking this dish while substantially reducing total cooking time. The creamy texture of frozen brown rice goes well while cutting down on cooking time, too. Try using any extra pot liquor to boost the nutritional power of your morning smoothie.

4 SERVINGS

1 medium bunch (10 oz/280 g) collard greens, stems removed

1 cup (240 ml) canned light unsweetened coconut milk

1 cup (140 g) finely chopped onion

¾ cup (115 g) chopped green bell pepper

½ cup (45 g) sliced green onions, white and green parts

1 Tbsp dried thyme

¼ tsp ground allspice

¼ tsp red chile flakes

Sea salt and freshly ground black pepper

1 can (15 oz/425 g) black beans, drained and rinsed

3 cups (585 g) frozen cooked long-grain brown rice

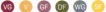

In a large saucepan, bring 2 cups (475 ml) water to a boil over high heat. Add the collard greens, pushing them into the water with a wooden spoon. Reduce the heat, cover, and simmer until the collards are still a bit tough, 6 minutes. Drain, reserving the cooking liquid. When the greens are cool enough to handle, chop, then set them aside.

In a large, heavy saucepan or small Dutch oven over medium-high heat, heat 2 Tbsp of the coconut milk. When the milk bubbles, add the onion and bell pepper and cook, stirring occasionally, until the onions have softened, 5 minutes.

Add the collard greens, green onions, thyme, allspice, and red chile flakes. Pour in the remaining coconut milk and 1½ cups (350 ml) of pot liquor from the greens. Reduce the heat and simmer, covered, until the greens are tender, 20 minutes, stirring 2 or 3 times. Add 1 tsp salt.

Add the beans and stir to combine them with the greens. Mix in the rice. Cover and cook for 5 minutes to warm the beans and thaw the rice. Adjust the seasoning with salt and pepper to taste. Cover and let the pot sit off the heat for 5 minutes to let the flavors marry. Serve in shallow, wide bowls.

Lemon Dal

In India, protein-rich dal, usually made with lentils, accompanies nearly every meal. Red lentils cook in less than thirty minutes. Do rinse them thoroughly to remove the fine dust they create by rubbing together. Lemon zest adds bright flavor and important phytonutrients found only in citrus's colorful outer peel. Dal, dark greens, and rice together make a sustaining vegan meal.

4 SERVINGS

⅔ cup (130 g) red lentils

1 Tbsp coconut oil or avocado oil

½ yellow onion, finely chopped

1 large clove garlic, minced

2 tsp peeled and grated fresh ginger

½ tsp ground turmeric

1 Tbsp tomato paste

2 cups (500 ml) low-sodium vegetable broth

1½ tsp grated lemon zest

Sea salt and freshly ground black pepper

¼ cup (10 g) chopped fresh cilantro

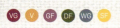

In a medium bowl, cover the lentils with cold water to a depth of 2 inches (5 cm). Swish with your hand, then drain the lentils. Repeat 3 or 4 times, until the drained water runs almost clear.

In a large saucepan over medium-high heat, heat the oil. Add the onion and cook, stirring occasionally, until softened, about 4 minutes. Mix in the garlic, ginger, and turmeric, and cook until fragrant, 30 seconds. Mix in the tomato paste until combined with the onion and spices, 30 seconds.

Add the lentils, broth, and 1 cup (240 ml) water. Bring to a boil over high heat, reduce the heat to medium-low, cover, and simmer until the lentils are soft but still have some texture, 25 minutes.

Off the heat, mix in the lemon zest. Season with salt and pepper. Ladle the dal into individual bowls, garnish with the cilantro, and serve right away.

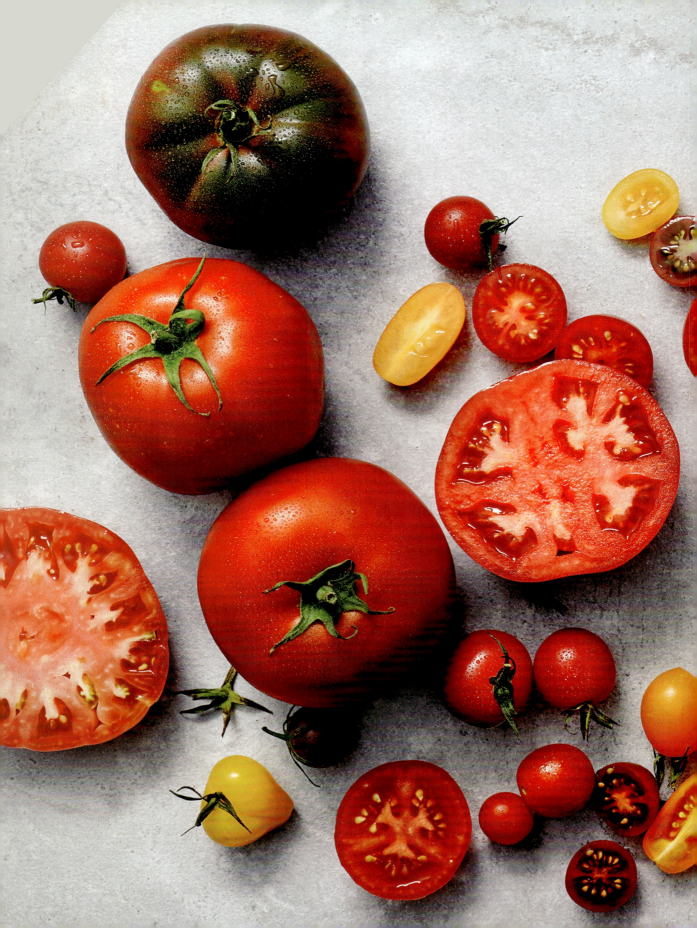

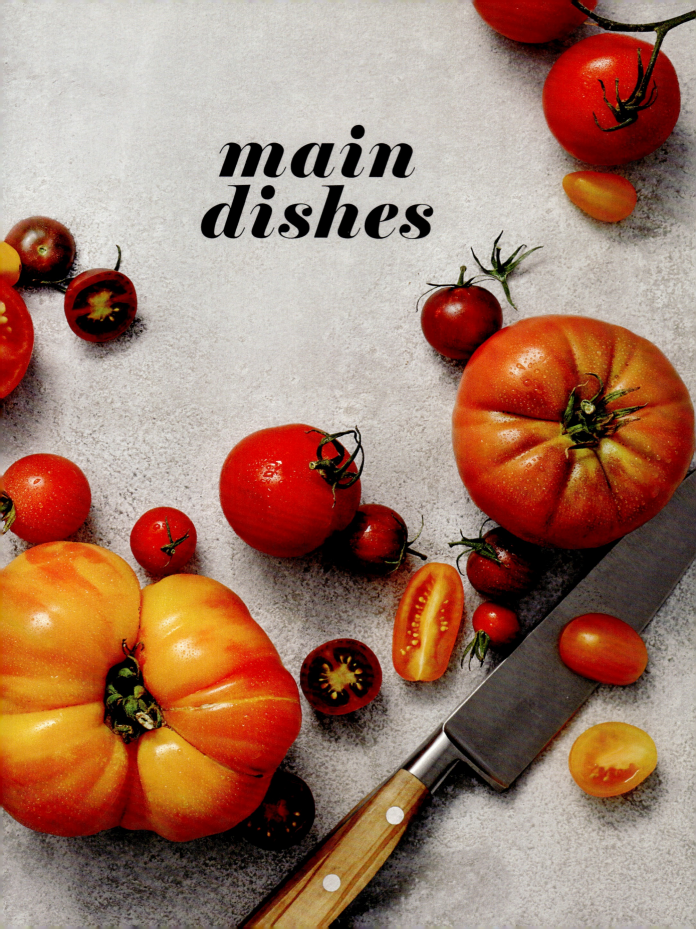

main dishes

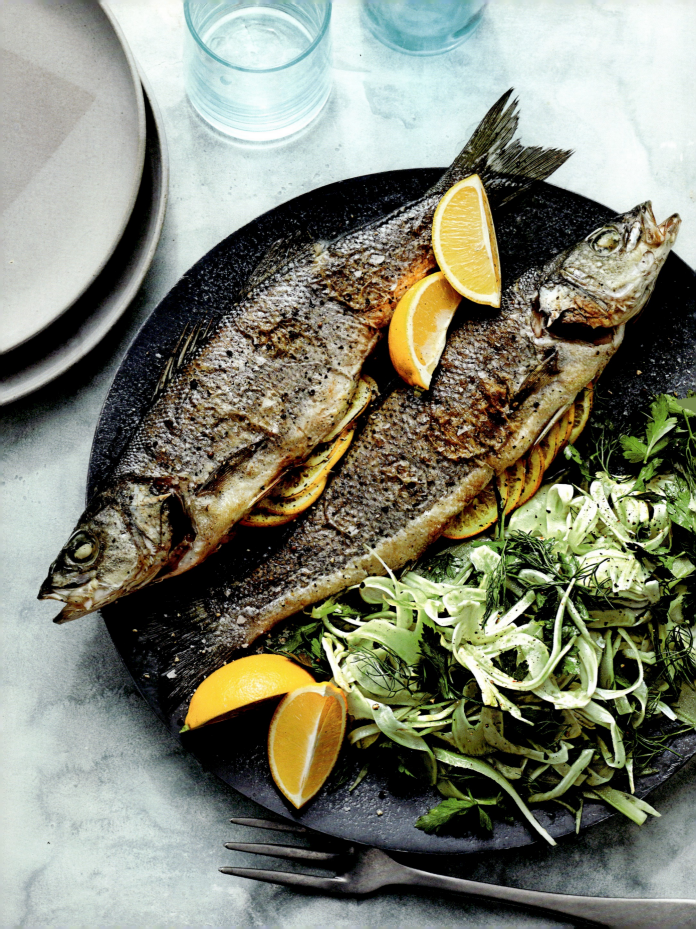

Whole Roasted Branzino with Meyer Lemon & Shaved Fennel

With its buttery, mild flavor, branzino, the Mediterranean sea bass also known as loup de mer luc, is complimented here by sweet-tart Meyer lemon and a fresh fennel salad. This dish's protein and antioxidants make it a good restorative meal after working out. It is also an excellent choice for hesitant fish eaters. The silky texture and gentle flavor of trout make it a fine substitute, if you wish.

2 SERVINGS

1 fennel bulb

½ cup (20 g) packed fresh flat-leaf parsley leaves, chopped

3 Tbsp extra-virgin olive oil

2 tsp white wine vinegar

Kosher salt and freshly ground black pepper

2 or 3 whole branzino (about ¾ lb/350 g each), cleaned

6 Tbsp (90 ml) olive oil

2 lemons, sliced

Position a rack in the upper third of the oven and preheat the oven to 400°F (200°C). Line a baking sheet with parchment paper.

Trim the fennel, reserving the fronds. Halve the bulb lengthwise and cut away the core if it seems tough. Using a mandoline or other hand slicer, thinly shave the fennel halves lengthwise (or quarter the bulb and shave with a vegetable peeler). Chop the fronds.

In a bowl, combine the shaved fennel, fennel fronds, parsley, olive oil, and vinegar and toss to coat well. Season to taste with salt and pepper and set aside at room temperature while you prepare the fish.

Rinse and dry the fish well, then place on the prepared pan. Drizzle 3 Tbsp of the oil over each fish and rub it all over, being sure to get into the cavity. Season the whole fish, inside and out, generously with salt and pepper. Lay the lemon slices in the cavity, overlapping them slightly.

Bake the fish for 10 minutes. The fish will turn slightly opaque and the lemons will wilt. Turn on the broiler to its highest setting and broil until the flesh of the fish is opaque when tested with a knife and the skin is crisp, about 5 minutes.

Serve with the fennel slaw and with extra lemon slices, if desired.

Seared Sea Bass with Miso Butter & Crispy Kale

Every element in this dish is rich in protein and provides an abundance of vitamins, making it a great choice in stressful times. Miso, made with fermented soybeans, aids digestion and helps boost the immune system.

4 SERVINGS

2 cups (120 g) stemmed and roughly torn kale leaves

2 Tbsp olive oil

Kosher salt and freshly ground black pepper

1 tsp paprika

4 Tbsp (60 g) unsalted butter

1 Tbsp white miso paste

4 skin-on sea bass fillets (about 6 oz/180 g each)

2 Tbsp avocado oil or coconut oil

Lemon wedges, for serving

Preheat the oven to 375°F (190°C). Top a baking sheet with a wire rack.

In a bowl, toss the kale with the olive oil to coat evenly. Season generously with salt and pepper. Arrange the kale in a single layer on the rack on the pan. Sprinkle the paprika evenly over the kale. Roast the kale until crisp, about 10 minutes, flipping the pieces once halfway through the cooking time. Set aside. Leave the oven on.

In a small saucepan over medium heat, melt the butter. Cook, stirring frequently, until it is browned and has a toasty, nutty smell, 4–6 minutes. Remove from the heat and stir in the miso. Set aside.

Pat the bass fillets dry and season with salt and pepper. In a nonstick frying pan over medium-high heat, heat the avocado oil. Add the fillets, skin-side down, and cook until the skin is crisp, about 5 minutes. Flip the fillets flesh-side down and sear until the fish is cooked through when tested with a knife tip, 5–7 minutes longer. For very thick fillets, flip back to skin-side down and finish in the preheated oven.

Divide the fillets among serving plates and spoon the miso butter over the top. Garnish with the kale chips and lemon wedges, and serve right away.

Pan-Seared Scallops with Sautéed Citrus

Citrus slices and freshly squeezed juice complement the richness of sea scallops. Blood oranges, in season from November to March, get their distinctive deep red flesh and berry-like flavor from anthocyanins, which are potent antioxidants. Better quality navel oranges have smaller, tighter navels. Whatever variety, oranges provide more than a day's worth of vitamin C, helpful for keeping colds at bay.

4 SERVINGS

2 each navel oranges and blood oranges

Sea salt and freshly ground black pepper

½ tsp ground cumin

1 lb (500 g) large sea scallops

1 Tbsp olive oil

2 tsp sherry vinegar

1 Tbsp unsalted butter

2 tsp chopped fresh cilantro

Cut one of each type of orange into thin rounds, and juice the others. Set aside.

In a small dish, combine a pinch each of salt and pepper with the cumin. Sprinkle the scallops with the seasoning mixture. In a frying pan over medium-high heat, heat the olive oil. Cook the scallops until browned on the bottom side, 1–2 minutes. Turn and cook on the other side until just firm to the touch and still a bit translucent in the center, 1–2 minutes longer. Transfer to a plate and keep warm.

Add the vinegar and reserved orange juice to the pan and cook until reduced by half, 1–2 minutes. Add the orange slices and cook for 1 minute. Remove from the heat and stir in the butter. Return the scallops along with any juices to the pan and stir to coat with the sauce.

Transfer to plates, top with the sauce and oranges, sprinkle with cilantro, and serve right away.

Fish Curry with Coconut, Potatoes & Peas

This golden curry has a coconut-milk base. Curry powder is a flavorful blend, usually combining eight or more antioxidant-rich spices, including turmeric. Using it saves time and lots of room on your spice rack. The blend known as Madras curry powder is perfect here. Keeping the peel on the potatoes adds flavor and retains the most nutritious part.

4 SERVINGS

2 Tbsp avocado oil or coconut oil

⅔ cup (80 g) finely chopped yellow onion

2 cloves garlic, each cut into 4 slices

2 tsp hot or mild curry powder

½ lb (250 g) small yellow-fleshed potatoes, halved or quartered

½ cup (125 ml) low-sodium chicken broth

½ tsp sea salt

1 lb (500 g) cod, cut into 8 pieces

⅔ cup (75 g) frozen peas

1 cup (250 ml) unsweetened light coconut milk

1 Tbsp fresh lemon juice

In a small Dutch oven over medium-high heat, heat the oil. When the oil shimmers, add the onion and cook until golden, about 7 minutes, stirring often towards the end. Add the garlic and curry powder, stirring to coat the onions. Cook until they are fragrant, 1–2 minutes.

Add the potatoes, stirring to coat them with the curry. Pour in the broth. Add the salt and ½ cup (125 ml) water, cover, and simmer until the potatoes are tender, 10–12 minutes.

Add the fish to the pot, placing the pieces in one layer. Add the peas and pour in the coconut milk. When the liquid returns to a simmer, reduce the heat and cook, covered, until the thickest pieces of fish are just opaque in the center, about 5 minutes.

Off the heat, add the lemon juice. Divide the curry among wide, shallow soup bowls. Serve right away.

 Choose organic potatoes, if possible, for this unpeeled use.

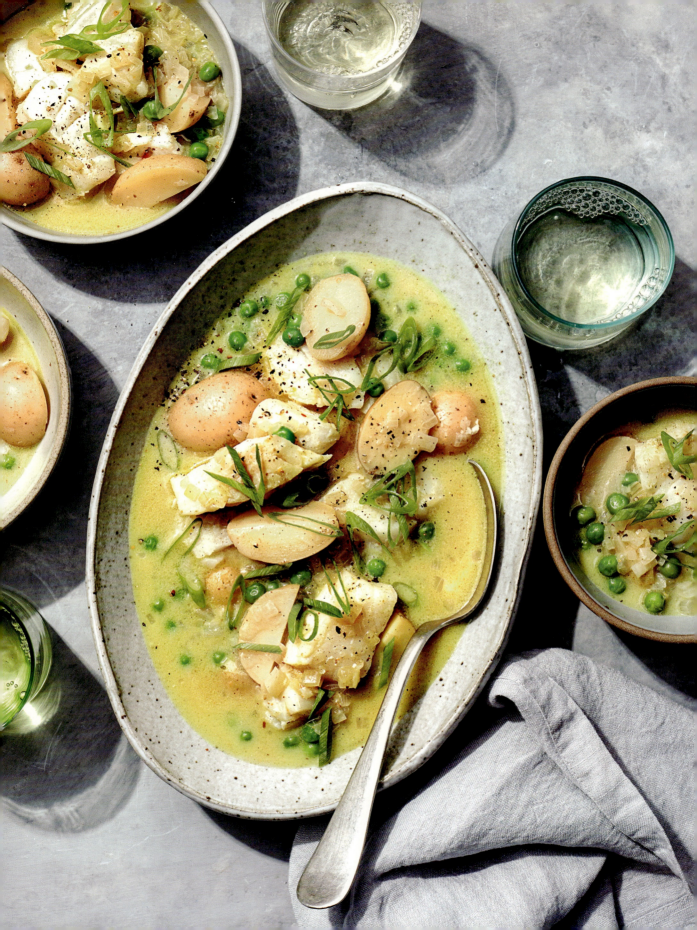

Roasted Salmon with Thyme Vinaigrette

Fresh wild Alaska salmon, an all-time favorite of fish lovers, starts its season in early spring. A salad of mixed baby greens is an ideal accompaniment to this omega-3-rich fatty fish. Smashed young potatoes (page 131) round out the meal perfectly. Be sure you leave their skins on to benefit most from their vitamin C, potassium, and fiber.

2 SERVINGS

½ Tbsp Dijon mustard

2 tsp Champagne vinegar or white wine vinegar

2 ½ Tbsp extra-virgin olive oil, plus more as needed

1 Tbsp minced shallot

2 tsp minced fresh thyme

Kosher salt and freshly ground black pepper

1 salmon fillet (about ¾ lb/350 g)

3 cups (90 g) mixed baby lettuces

Preheat the oven to 425°F (220°C). Put the mustard in a medium bowl and whisk in the vinegar. Gradually whisk in 2 ½ Tbsp olive oil. Stir in the shallot and thyme. Season the vinaigrette to taste with salt and pepper.

Brush a small baking dish with oil. Place the salmon in the dish, skin-side down. Spoon half of the vinaigrette over the salmon. Let marinate for up to 1 hour.

Roast the salmon until almost cooked through, about 15 minutes. Let it rest while you prepare the salad.

Add the lettuces to the bowl with the remaining vinaigrette and toss. Divide the salad between serving plates. Cut the salmon in half and put one piece alongside the salad on each plate. Serve right away.

TIP *This recipe easily doubles to serve four, or provides leftovers for a salmon salad dinner the next night. For convenience, make the vinaigrette a day ahead of time. You can also double or triple the dressing to have extra to use on salads later in the week.*

Seared Trout with Fresh Herb Salad

Sautéing fish skin-side down in a covered skillet is a great technique that yields crisp skin and tender flesh without the need for any flour—a boon for the gluten-free diner. A mustard and lemon vinaigrette both seasons the fish and dresses the salad.

4 SERVINGS

1 ½ lb (680 g) fingerling potatoes, halved lengthwise

2 Tbsp plus ½ cup (125 ml) extra-virgin olive oil

Kosher salt and freshly ground black pepper

1 tsp Dijon mustard

¼ cup (60 ml) fresh lemon juice

3 green onions, white and pale green parts, 1 minced and 2 thinly sliced

4 trout fillets (5–6 oz/ 150–180 g each)

2 cups (70 g) baby salad greens

2 cups (60 g) fresh flat-leaf parsley leaves

1 large bunch fresh dill, roughly chopped (about ½ cup/30 g)

½ cup (15 g) packed fresh basil leaves

DF SF

Preheat the oven to 425°F (220°C). In a large bowl, toss the potatoes with 1 Tbsp of the olive oil. Sprinkle with salt and pepper and toss to coat. Arrange the potatoes on a large rimmed baking sheet, cut-side down. Roast until browned on the cut side and tender, about 25 minutes.

Meanwhile, in a small bowl, combine the mustard and lemon juice. Slowly whisk in the ½ cup (125 ml) olive oil to make a vinaigrette. Stir in the minced green onion, then season to taste with salt and pepper. Transfer 2 Tbsp of the vinaigrette to a small bowl and brush over the flesh side of the fish. In a salad bowl, combine the greens, parsley, dill, basil leaves, and two-thirds of the sliced green onions.

In a 12-inch (30-cm) nonstick frying pan over medium-high heat, heat the remaining 1 Tbsp oil. Add the fish, skin-side down. Cover the pan and cook the fish without turning until springy to the touch, about 5 minutes.

Dress the salad with vinaigrette to taste and toss well. Divide the salad among serving plates. Top with the fish, and then drizzle the fish with a little more vinaigrette. Arrange the potatoes alongside, and serve right away.

TIP *This recipe is just as good with wild salmon, halibut, orArctic char. There will be plenty of vinaigrette left to use another night on a salad or chicken.*

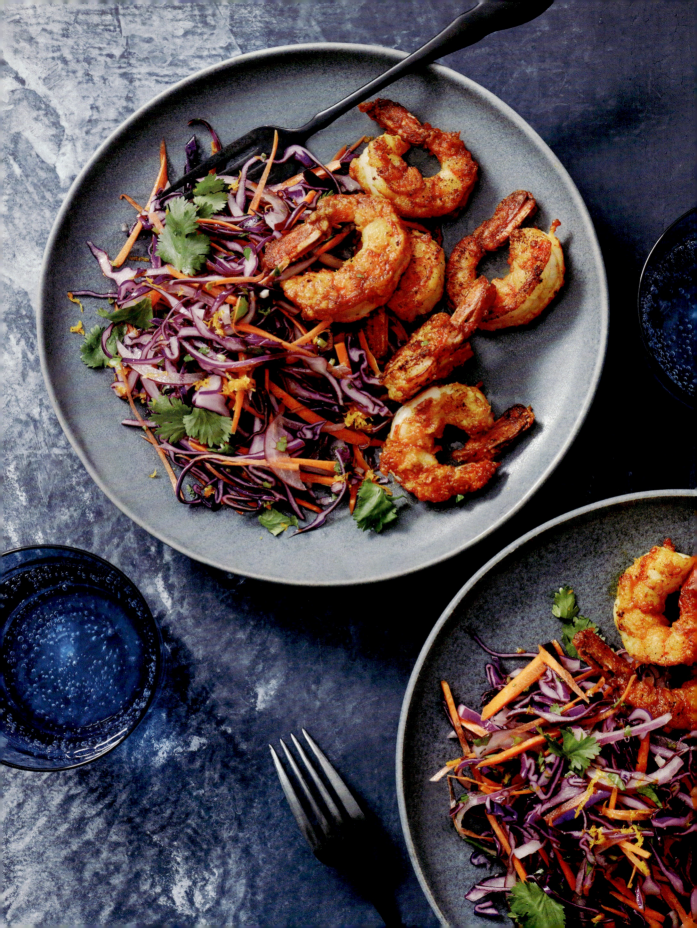

Turmeric Shrimp with Red Cabbage & Carrot Slaw

Here, garlicky, turmeric-coated shrimp—low in calories and high in protein—are complemented by a citrus-dressed slaw rich in micronutrients. Be sure the turmeric you use is fresh to get maximum flavor and antioxidant benefits.

6 SERVINGS

FOR THE SLAW

½ cup (125 ml) fresh orange juice, plus grated zest of 2 large oranges

3 Tbsp white wine vinegar

¾ cup (180 ml) avocado oil or extra-virgin olive oil

2 cloves garlic, minced

½ tsp Tabasco or other hot pepper sauce

½ tsp ground cumin

Salt and freshly ground pepper

4 oz (120 g) shredded red cabbage (2 cups)

2 large carrots, peeled and julienned, shaved, or spiralized

¼ cup (40 g) finely chopped red onion

3 Tbsp chopped fresh cilantro

¼ cup (30 g) all-purpose flour

1 tsp ground turmeric

½ tsp chili powder

Sea salt

1 ½ lb (680 g) jumbo shrimp, peeled and deveined, tails intact

2 Tbsp avocado oil or coconut oil

4 cloves garlic, smashed

1 Tbsp unsalted butter

To make the slaw, in a large bowl, whisk together the orange juice, vinegar, avocado oil, garlic, Tabasco, cumin, ½ tsp salt, and ¼ tsp pepper until well combined. Add the cabbage, carrots, onion, and half each of the cilantro and orange zest and stir until combined. Cover and refrigerate for at least 1 hour and up to 2 hours so the vegetables wilt slightly and the flavors marry.

In a wide, shallow bowl, stir together the flour, turmeric, chili powder, and ½ tsp salt. Add the shrimp and toss to coat lightly but evenly.

In a large frying pan over medium-high heat, heat the 2 Tbsp avocado oil (use 2 smaller pans if needed to prevent crowding). Add the garlic and cook, stirring continuously, until golden brown, 45–60 seconds. Using a slotted spoon, remove and discard the garlic.

Return the pan to medium heat. Add the butter and, when the foam subsides, add half the shrimp in a single layer and cook for 1 minute, then turn and continue to cook until pink and firm, 1–2 minutes longer. (You will need to start turning the shrimp that were added first as soon as you add the last one; keep track of the order so you don't overcook them.) Transfer the shrimp to a platter and keep warm while you cook the remaining shrimp.

Serve the shrimp with the slaw on the side, sprinkled with the remaining cilantro and orange zest.

Fish Tacos with Broccoli Slaw & Lime Crema

This is a fresh take on fish tacos: spice-coated tuna sautéed until crisp on the outside but slightly pink inside, a slaw made with sweet shredded broccoli, and everything topped with a creamy sauce spiked with fresh lime. It's the complete package of proteins, vitamins, and omega-3 fats. If you prefer, use gluten-free tortillas.

4 SERVINGS

FOR THE BROCCOLI SLAW

4 cups (8 oz/250 g) prepared broccoli coleslaw (about half of a 16-oz/500-g bag)

¼ cup (45 g) minced red onion

¼ cup (15 g) minced fresh cilantro

1 Tbsp plus 1 tsp fresh lime juice

1 serrano chile, seeded and minced

Salt and freshly ground pepper

FOR THE LIME CREMA

6 Tbsp (90 ml) heavy cream

6 Tbsp (90 g) sour cream

1 ½ tsp finely grated lime zest

2 ½ tsp fresh lime juice

1 lb (500 g) albacore tuna, cut into ¾-inch (2 cm) cubes

¾ tsp ancho chile powder

¼ tsp each ground cumin and ground coriander

2 Tbsp olive oil

8–10 taco-sized tortillas (5–6 inches/14–15 cm in diameter)

1 large avocado, halved, pitted, and sliced

In a large bowl, combine the broccoli slaw, onion, cilantro, the 1 Tbsp plus 1 tsp lime juice, and the minced serrano. Toss to combine. Season to taste with salt and pepper. Let the slaw stand while preparing the sauce and fish.

In a small bowl, whisk together the cream and sour cream, then add the lime zest, lime juice, and a pinch of salt and whisk again. Set aside.

In a medium bowl, mix the tuna cubes, chile powder, cumin, and coriander. Sprinkle with salt and pepper. In a large frying pan over medium-high heat, heat the oil. Add the fish and sauté until brown on the outside but still pink inside, about 2 minutes. Transfer the fish to a bowl.

Meanwhile, to toast the tortillas, place them one at a time directly over a gas burner or in a heated dry skillet and cook until a few brown spots appear, about 20 seconds on each side. Keep warm in a tortilla warmer or wrapped in aluminum foil.

Set the fish, slaw, crema, avocado, and tortillas out on the table and let diners assemble their own tacos.

Pan-Roasted Mussels with Fennel Seed, Saffron & Basil

Mussels are versatile, fast cooking, and contain a super combination of protein, omega-3s, and minerals. They roast beautifully in a cast-iron pan in a hot oven, which surrounds them with heat and helps them cook quickly and evenly. Most mussels are sustainably farmed and easy to clean but do make sure they are free of grit so you can enjoy sopping up their aromatic broth with grilled bread.

4 SERVINGS

2 lb (1 kg) large mussels

2 Tbsp unsalted butter

2 Tbsp olive oil

4 cloves garlic, minced

Pinch of red chile flakes

½ cup (125 ml) dry white vermouth or wine

1 tsp fennel seeds, toasted

Pinch of saffron threads, toasted, and dissolved in 1 Tbsp hot water

⅓ cup (20 g) finely shredded fresh basil leaves

Kosher salt

GF SF

Preheat the oven to 400°F (200°C). Rinse the mussels under cold running water and debeard them if needed. Discard any that don't close to the touch.

In a large cast-iron frying pan or ovenproof sauté pan over medium heat, melt the butter with the olive oil until the butter foams and subsides. Add the garlic and red chile flakes and sauté until fragrant, about 1 minute. Add the mussels, vermouth, fennel seeds, and the saffron mixture. Raise the heat to high and sauté for 30 seconds. Transfer the pan to the oven and roast until the mussels open, 4–6 minutes.

Remove from the oven and discard any mussels that failed to open. Sprinkle the mussels with the basil and season to taste with salt. Serve right away in the pan.

Roasted Caesar Salad with Salmon

Yes, roasted! Also roasting the lettuce adds a smoky flavor that complements the brightness of the Caesar dressing. The crisp, compact leaves of romaine lettuce hearts can take the heat of roasting without going limp. For a leaner dish, swap out the salmon for shrimp; for a more mineral-rich and vegetarian version, replace the salmon with grilled tofu.

4–6 SERVINGS

4 center-cut wild salmon fillets (about 6 oz/180 g each)

3 Tbsp olive oil

Sea salt and freshly ground black pepper

3 anchovies in olive oil

1 clove garlic

1 tsp dried mustard

Juice of 1 lemon

2 hearts of romaine or 2 heads Little Gem lettuce, leaves separated

¼ cup (1 oz/30 g) freshly grated Parmesan cheese

Preheat the oven to 425°F (220°C). Line a baking sheet with parchment paper. Place the salmon on one end of the prepared pan. Brush the salmon with 1 Tbsp of the oil and season with salt and pepper. Roast for 5 minutes.

Finely chop the anchovies and garlic on a cutting board and sprinkle with ½ tsp salt. Use the side of your knife to make a paste and transfer to a mixing bowl. Stir in the mustard and the lemon juice. Whisk in the remaining 2 Tbsp olive oil and season to taste with more salt and pepper.

Pull the salmon out of the oven and place the hearts of romaine on the other end of the baking sheet. Brush with a good amount of the dressing and return the pan to the oven. Roast just until the salmon is opaque throughout and the top of the lettuce begins to char, 7–10 minutes. Remove the pan from the oven. Sprinkle the lettuce with the Parmesan cheese.

Arrange the lettuce leaves on a platter or divide among dinner plates. Top with the salmon and drizzle with the remaining dressing. Serve right away.

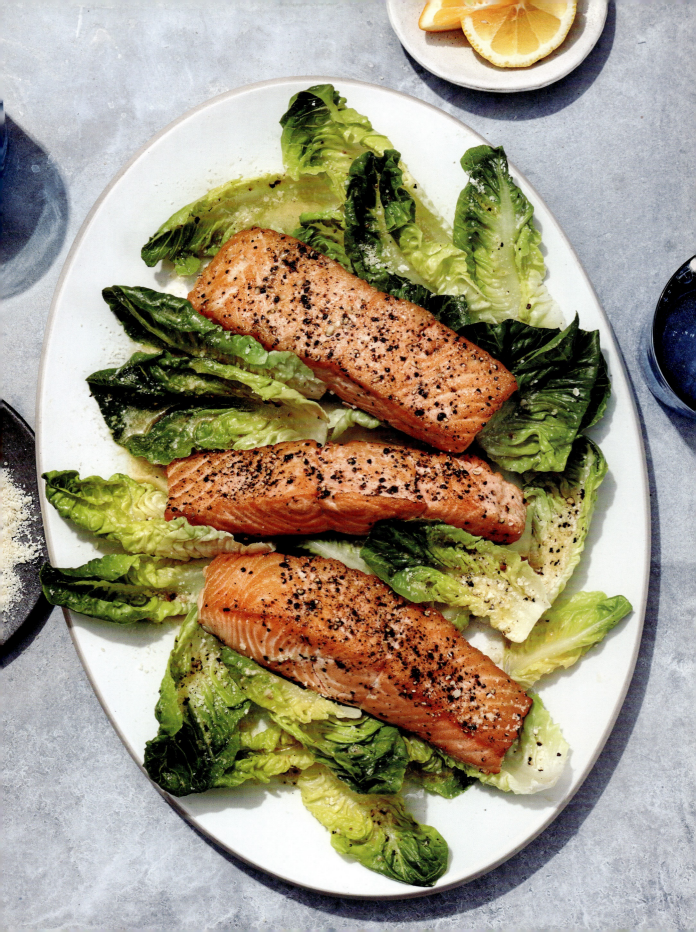

Moroccan Roast Chicken & Vegetables

A quartet of familiar spices brings the aromatic flavors of Morocco to this complete meal in one. Those who struggle to fit in the recommended five servings a day of vegetables will love the cauliflower bathed in spices and the flavor of the chicken. The work is done once the bird is in the oven, freeing you to enjoy a pre-dinner cocktail or mocktail.

4 SERVINGS

5 Tbsp (75 ml) olive oil, plus more for greasing

1 chicken (about 5 lb/2.5 kg)

Kosher salt and freshly ground black pepper

2 Tbsp plus 1 ½ tsp sweet paprika

1 ½ tsp ground cumin

¾ tsp red chile flakes

¾ tsp ground cinnamon

1 lemon

2 small orange-fleshed sweet potatoes (about ¾ lb/350 g total weight), unpeeled

1 lb (500 g) cauliflower, cut into 1-inch (2.5-cm) florets

1 red onion, cut into 8 wedges

Preheat the oven to 450°F (230°C). Grease a large, heavy rimmed baking sheet. Pull out and discard the fat and giblets from the main cavity in the chicken. Pat the chicken dry with paper towels. Starting at the edge of the main cavity, slide a finger under the skin over each breast half, making pockets. Rub 1 Tbsp salt all over the chicken and in the main cavity. Sprinkle generously with black pepper. Tie the legs together, if desired.

In a small bowl, mix the paprika, cumin, red chile flakes, and cinnamon. Set aside 2 ½ tsp of the spice mixture for the vegetables. Finely grate the zest from the lemon, cut the lemon into quarters, and mix the zest into the remaining spices. Mix in 2 Tbsp of the olive oil to make a paste. Spread some paste inside the main cavity and under the skin; rub the rest of the paste all over the outside of the chicken. Insert the lemon quarters into the main cavity. Place the chicken in the center of the prepared pan and roast for 40–45 minutes.

Meanwhile, cut the sweet potatoes in half crosswise; quarter each piece lengthwise, forming wedges. Combine the sweet potatoes, cauliflower, and onion in a bowl. Add the remaining 3 Tbsp oil and toss to coat. Add the reserved spice mixture. Sprinkle with ½ tsp each salt and pepper, and toss to coat.

After the chicken has roasted for 35 minutes, remove from the oven. Tilt the baking sheet and spoon off most of the fat. Arrange the chicken in the center of the pan and spoon the vegetables around the bird. Continue roasting until an instant-read thermometer inserted into the thickest part of a thigh registers 165°F (74°C), about 30 minutes longer. (The bird will take longer to roast if the legs have been tied together). If the skin is getting too dark, reduce the oven temperature to 425°F (220°C). Transfer to a platter and let rest for 10 minutes. Carve the chicken, and serve right away with the vegetables.

Chicken Tostadas with Radish Slaw

Vitamin-rich radishes are routinely part of the salsa and condiment spreads available at the best taquerias. Use them here as part of a fresh topping for earthy chicken tostadas. Achiote paste, a popular Yucatecan seasoning made from ground annatto seeds, is available at Mexican groceries and well-stocked supermarkets, or online.

6 SERVINGS

FOR THE CHICKEN

⅔ cup (160 ml) fresh orange juice

3 Tbsp fresh lime juice

3 Tbsp achiote paste

1 small yellow onion, chopped

2 cloves garlic, chopped

½ tsp dried oregano

2 lb (1 kg) boneless, skinless chicken thighs

Kosher salt and freshly ground black pepper

FOR THE RADISH SLAW

About 18 radishes, trimmed, halved, and thinly sliced

2 green onions, white and pale green parts, thinly sliced

⅓ cup (10 g) fresh cilantro, chopped

1 Tbsp fresh lime juice

Corn oil, for frying

12 corn tortillas, 4 inches (10 cm) in diameter

¾ cup (3 oz/90 g) crumbled cotija cheese

2 large avocados, halved, pitted, and sliced

To prepare the chicken, in a heavy Dutch oven, stir together the orange juice, lime juice, and achiote paste until the achiote paste is smooth. Add the onion, garlic, and oregano and mix well. Add the chicken thighs and turn to coat evenly. Sprinkle the chicken with salt. Cover, place over medium heat, bring to a simmer, then reduce the heat to low and cook, stirring occasionally, until the sauce has thickened and the chicken is opaque throughout when pierced with a knife tip, about 40 minutes. Uncover and continue to simmer until the sauce is very thick and the chicken begins to fall apart and catch on the bottom of the pan, about 10 minutes.

Remove from the heat and let cool slightly, then shred the chicken. Season with salt and pepper.

To make the radish slaw, in a small bowl, combine the radishes, green onions, cilantro, and lime juice and toss to mix. Season with salt. Pour oil to a depth of 1 inch (2.5 cm) into a deep, heavy frying pan and warm over medium-high heat until almost smoking. One at a time, add the tortillas and cook, turning once with tongs, until crisp and golden, 1–2 minutes. As each tortilla is ready, transfer it to paper towels to drain, then sprinkle lightly with salt.

Arrange 2 tortillas side by side on each individual plate. Top the tortillas with the chicken, dividing it equally, and then spoon the radish slaw evenly over the chicken. Top the tostadas evenly with the cheese and the avocado slices, and serve right away.

GF SF

Roast Chicken with Heirloom Tomato & Sourdough Panzanella

This Mediterranean take on roast chicken is perfect for casual weekend entertaining or a family dinner packed with protein, micronutrients, and good carbs. It's also an excellent way to recycle day-old bread by turning it into generously large croutons bathed in olive oil.

6-8 SERVINGS

1 lb (500 g) sourdough bread, torn into 2-inch (5-cm) pieces

5 Tbsp (75 ml) olive oil, plus more for rubbing

Kosher salt and freshly ground black pepper

1 whole chicken, 4–5 lb (about 2 kg), cut into 8 serving pieces

2 ½ lb (1.2 kg) assorted heirloom tomatoes, cored and roughly chopped

½ cup (70 g) pine nuts

1 small shallot, minced

2 cloves garlic, minced

½ tsp Dijon mustard

2 tsp white wine vinegar

4 Tbsp (60 g) butter, cut into 4 equal pieces

1 cup (225 g) cherry tomatoes, halved

½ cup (15 g) packed fresh basil leaves, stacked and thinly sliced, plus whole leaves for garnish

Preheat the oven to 350°F (180°C). Put the sourdough bread in a large bowl, drizzle with 3 Tbsp of the oil, toss, and season with salt and pepper. Spread in a single layer on a baking sheet and bake until golden, about 15 minutes. Set aside to cool completely. Raise the oven temperature to 450°F (230°C).

Arrange the chicken pieces on a second baking sheet. Rub generously with olive oil and season with salt and pepper. Roast until an instant-read thermometer inserted into the thickest part of a thigh registers 175°F (80°C), 40–50 minutes. For crispy skin, move the pan to the upper third of the oven, turn the oven setting to broil, and broil the chicken for 3 minutes.

Meanwhile, in a colander set over a large bowl, toss the heirloom tomatoes with 2 tsp salt. Let stand, stirring occasionally, until the juices release and drain into the bowl, about 15 minutes.

In a small frying pan over medium heat, heat the remaining 2 Tbsp olive oil. Add the pine nuts and cook, stirring occasionally, until toasted, 3–5 minutes. Pour onto a small plate to cool.

Transfer the colander with the tomatoes to the sink. Add the shallot, garlic, mustard, and vinegar to the tomato juices in the bowl and set aside.

Remove the chicken from the oven, transfer to a plate, and keep warm. Add the butter to the baking sheet with the pan drippings and return it to the oven until the butter melts, about 1 minute. Add the butter mixture to the bowl of tomato juices and whisk well. Add the bread, drained tomatoes, cherry tomatoes, basil, and pine nuts and mix well. Season to taste with salt and pepper. Let sit until the bread has absorbed the liquids, about 5 minutes.

Transfer the panzanella to a platter and top with the chicken pieces. Garnish with basil leaves and serve right away.

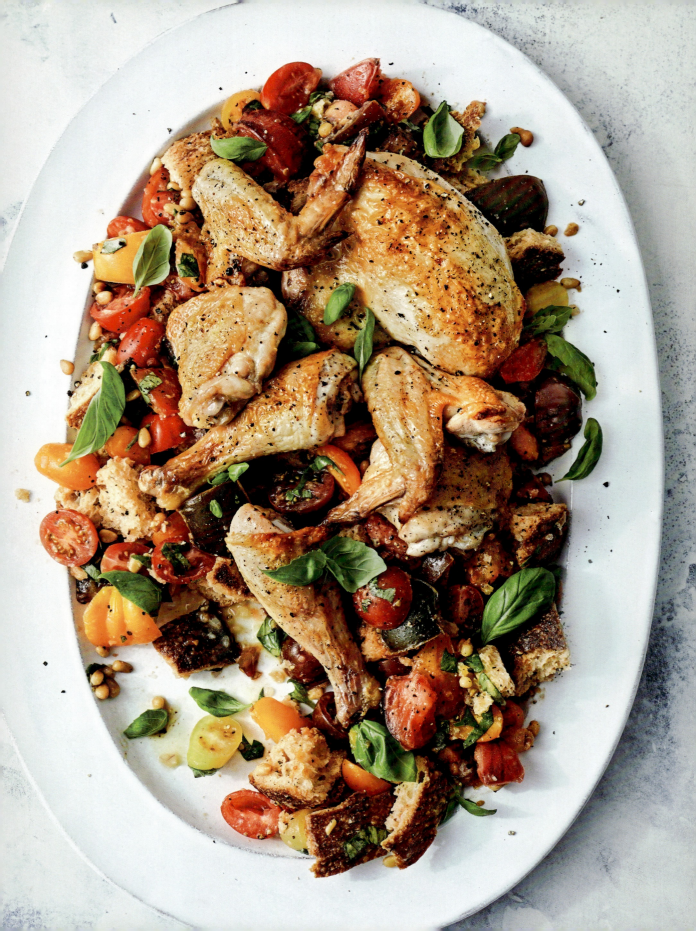

Chicken Shawarma
with Peppers & Tahini

Warmly spiced chicken and vegetables make a wonderful Middle Eastern dinner, especially when served with homemade tahini sauce. If you are short on time, replace the tahini sauce with store-bought hummus—both offer a satisfying trio of fiber, healthy fat, and protein.

4–6 SERVINGS

6 Tbsp (90 ml) olive oil

Juice of 1 lemon

2 cloves garlic, chopped

1 ½ tsp ground cumin

¾ tsp ground turmeric

¾ tsp paprika

Kosher salt and freshly ground black pepper

1 ½ lb (680 g) boneless, skinless chicken breasts, cut into ½-inch (12-mm) slices

1 red and 1 yellow bell pepper, seeded and sliced into ½-inch-thick (12-mm) slices

1 red onion, halved and sliced into ½-inch-thick (12-mm) slices

FOR THE TAHINI SAUCE

1 clove garlic, roughly chopped

½ cup (120 g) tahini

Juice of 1 lemon

½ tsp ground cumin

½ cup (125 ml) warm water

6 pieces lavash or whole-wheat pita bread, warmed (optional)

In a large bowl, whisk together ¼ cup (60 ml) of the olive oil, the lemon juice, garlic, cumin, turmeric, paprika, 1 tsp salt, and ½ tsp pepper. Add the chicken and toss to coat. Cover and refrigerate for at least 2 hours and up to overnight.

Preheat the oven to 400°F (200°C). Line a baking sheet with aluminum foil. Remove the chicken from the marinade and place in a single layer on one end of the prepared pan.

In another bowl, toss together the bell peppers, onion, and the remaining 2 Tbsp olive oil. Place the vegetables in a single layer on the other end of the pan. Season the chicken and vegetables with salt and pepper. Roast, stirring once, until the chicken is opaque throughout and the vegetables are fork tender, 25–30 minutes.

Meanwhile, prepare the tahini sauce: In a food processor or blender, combine the garlic, tahini, lemon juice, cumin, and ¼ tsp salt and purée until well blended. Add the warm water and purée until smooth. Adjust the seasoning with salt.

Fill the lavash, if using, with the chicken and vegetables, drizzle with the tahini sauce, and serve right away.

Mustard Dill Turkey Burgers

*When you're cutting down on saturated fat but crave a good burger, turn to turkey.
Using ground turkey that's 93 percent lean provides enough fat for a juicy burger
with a modest amount of saturated fat. For an umami boost, top your burger with
sautéed mushrooms seasoned with soy sauce or gluten-free tamari.*

4 SERVINGS

⅓ cup (75 ml) olive-oil mayonnaise

5 Tbsp (75 g) Dijon mustard

5 Tbsp (⅓ cup/13 g) minced fresh dill

1 Tbsp plus 1 tsp fresh lemon juice

Kosher salt and freshly ground black pepper

4 cups (8 oz/250 g) prepared coleslaw mix (about half of a 16-oz/500-g bag)

3 green onions, minced

1 ¼ lb (570 g) ground turkey, preferably dark meat

Olive oil

4 toasted whole-wheat buns, or Olive Oil Mashed Potatoes (page 185) mixed with 2 Tbsp chopped fresh dill

In a small bowl, combine the mayonnaise, 3 Tbsp of the mustard, 2 Tbsp of the dill, and the 1 tsp lemon juice to make a sauce. Season to taste with salt and pepper.

In a large bowl, combine the coleslaw mix, ¼ cup (60 ml) of the sauce, the remaining 1 Tbsp lemon juice, and one-third of the green onions and toss to coat. Season to taste with salt and pepper.

In another large bowl, combine the ground turkey, remaining 2 Tbsp mustard, 3 Tbsp of the dill, the remaining green onions, ¾ tsp salt, and a generous amount of pepper. Mix gently. Form the mixture into 4 patties, each about ½ inch (12 mm) thick. Using your thumb, make an indentation in the center of each patty.

Heat a large frying pan over medium heat; brush with oil. Add the patties and cook until browned and cooked through in the center, about 5 minutes per side.

Place the bun bottoms on or spoon the potatoes in the center of serving plates. Top each with a patty and a spoonful of sauce. Spoon the coleslaw on top of the patty or alongside the potatoes, place the bun top, if using, over the slaw, and serve right away.

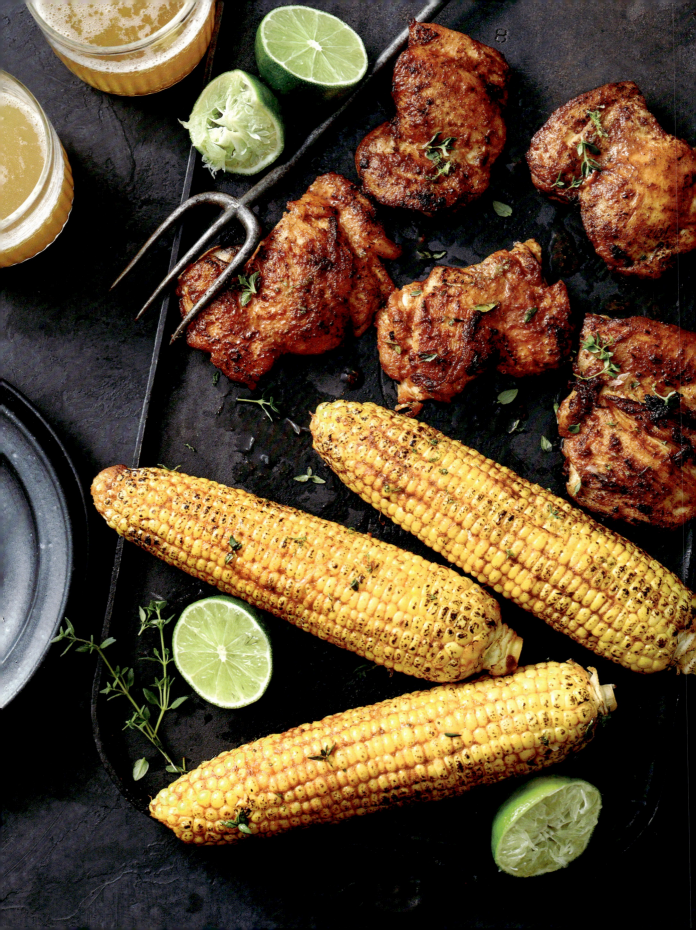

Grilled Chicken & Corn with Smoked Paprika Rub

Here, familiar chicken breasts and fresh corn are transformed with vibrant smoked paprika and fresh lime juice. Cooking them on the grill heightens the smoky flavor. Serve with a green salad to round out the vitamins and minerals, and finish the summery meal with sliced grilled peaches for a deliciously nutritious dessert (page 170).

4 SERVINGS

1 Tbsp smoked paprika

1 Tbsp ground cumin

3 Tbsp olive oil

3 Tbsp fresh lime juice

1 ¼–1 ½ lb (about 600 g) chicken breast cutlets

4 ears corn, husked

Kosher salt and freshly ground black pepper

1 ½ Tbsp grated lime zest

1 ½ Tbsp minced fresh thyme

In a small bowl, combine the paprika and cumin. Gradually mix in the olive oil and lime juice. Place the chicken and corn on a large baking sheet. Brush on all sides with the paprika mixture, and then sprinkle with salt and pepper.

Prepare a grill for direct-heat cooking over high heat (see Tip). Oil the grill grate. Add the corn to the grill rack, cover, and cook, turning frequently, until it starts to brown in spots and is almost tender, about 10 minutes. Add the chicken to the grill rack, cover, and cook until the chicken is springy to the touch and cooked through, about 3–5 minutes per side. Transfer the chicken and corn to a platter.

Sprinkle with lime zest and thyme, and serve right away.

TIP *In the event of inclement weather, the chicken is equally good sautéed. In that case, boil the corn, and season it after cooking. Leftover chicken makes great sandwiches, or you can cut up the chicken, cut the kernels from the corn ears, and add them both to a salad.*

Turkey Meatloaf with Mushroom Gravy

With cremini mushrooms in both the meatloaf and its gravy, this recipe delivers a double dose of their umami-rich flavor. Mushrooms help boost your immune system, an excellent idea during the cold months when you crave meatloaf most. The large baking pan allows room around the meatloaf for the mushrooms that will be the gravy base to soak up extra flavor.

6 SERVINGS

2 Tbsp avocado oil or coconut oil

8 oz (250 g) sliced cremini mushrooms

1 Tbsp dried thyme

½ cup (60 g) finely chopped onion

3 cloves garlic, finely chopped

1 Tbsp Worcestershire sauce

16–19 oz (500–540 g) ground turkey (93 percent lean)

1 slice soft whole-wheat bread, torn into ½-inch (12-mm) pieces

1 Tbsp tomato paste

1 Tbsp brown mustard

1 large egg

Sea salt and freshly ground black pepper

1 cup (250 ml) low-sodium beef broth

1 tsp unbleached all-purpose flour

In a medium frying pan over medium-high heat, heat the oil. Add the mushrooms and half the thyme and cook until the mushrooms look wet, 5 minutes. Add the onion, garlic, and Worcestershire sauce and cook, stirring occasionally, until the pan is nearly dry, 3 minutes.

On a cutting board, coarsely chop the cooked mushrooms. Place half the chopped mushrooms in a large mixing bowl. Set the rest aside.

To the bowl with the mushrooms, add the turkey, bread, tomato paste, mustard, egg, the remaining thyme, ½ tsp salt, and ¼ tsp pepper and mix with a fork until well combined. Coat a 13 x 9 x 2–inch (33 x 23 x 5–cm) baking pan with oil spray. Add the meat and shape into a 9 x 4–inch (23 x 10–cm) loaf.

Bake the meatloaf, tented loosely with foil, for 30 minutes. Uncover and add the remaining mushrooms and half the beef broth to the pan. Bake, uncovered, until an instant-read thermometer inserted into the center of the meatloaf registers 160°F (71°C). Let the meatloaf sit for 5 minutes, then transfer it to a serving plate.

Pour the contents of the baking pan into a medium saucepan. Add the flour and remaining broth and cook over medium heat, stirring, until the gravy thickens, about 3 minutes. Season with salt and pepper to taste. Slice the meatloaf and serve, accompanied by the gravy.

Pan-Roasted Turkey Cutlets with Lemon, Capers & White Wine

Turkey cutlets served with a lemon and white wine pan sauce make a healthy weeknight dinner with a touch of elegance. Pounding the cutlets tenderizes them and helps them cook quickly and evenly. Lightly flouring the lean turkey helps keep it juicy; for a gluten-free option, arrowroot powder makes a light coating and thickens the pan sauce. Replace the wine with a quarter cup (60 ml) of lemon juice, if you wish; in this variation, the sauce will thicken more quickly.

4 SERVINGS

4 turkey cutlets, about 1 lb (500 g) total weight

¼ cup (30 g) unbleached all-purpose flour or arrowroot powder

Sea salt and freshly ground black pepper

2 Tbsp extra-virgin olive oil

¼ cup (60 ml) dry white wine, such as sauvignon blanc

2 Tbsp fresh lemon juice

½ cup (125 ml) low-sodium chicken broth

1 Tbsp small capers, rinsed and drained

8 thin lemon slices, for garnish (optional)

Place each turkey cutlet between 2 sheets of plastic wrap and pound to an even thickness of ⅜ inch (1 cm).

On a plate, combine the flour with ½ tsp salt and ⅛ tsp pepper.

In a large frying pan over medium-high heat, heat 1 Tbsp of the olive oil. Working quickly, dredge a turkey cutlet in the seasoned flour, coating it lightly on both sides. Shake off any excess flour, then add the turkey to the pan. Repeat with the second cutlet. Cook until the cutlets are lightly browned on the bottom side, about 3 minutes. Turn and cook until the cutlets are brown on the second side and white in the center, about 2 minutes. Transfer the turkey to a serving plate and cover loosely with foil to keep warm.

Add the remaining 1 Tbsp oil to the pan. Flour and cook the remaining 2 cutlets.

After removing the last cutlet, pour the wine and lemon juice into the pan. Using a wooden spoon, scrape up any browned bits from the pan bottom. Add the broth. Raise the heat to high and boil until the sauce is reduced to ¼ cup (60 ml) and is golden brown and slightly thickened. Spoon the hot pan sauce over the turkey. Sprinkle on the capers. Top with the lemon slices, if using. Serve right away.

Shaking Beef with Spinach

Vietnamese bo luc lac—tender beef seared until crusty and served with a generous salad—makes a complete one-dish meal. It turns dinner into an occasion while requiring minimal hands-on time. The vinegar-marinated onions contain acid that helps your body absorb the iron in the spinach. The dish's name comes from shaking the pan to release the meat as it cooks.

4 SERVINGS

FOR THE MARINADE

4 tsp low-sodium soy sauce

1 ½ Tbsp brown rice miso

1 tsp fish sauce

3 Tbsp minced garlic

2 Tbsp brown sugar

¼ tsp freshly ground black pepper

1 ½ lb (680 g) rib eye steak, cut into 1-inch (2.5-cm) cubes

2 Tbsp red wine vinegar

2 Tbsp low-sodium soy sauce

1 Tbsp sugar

⅔ cup (70 g) thinly sliced red onion crescents

4 cups (4 oz/120 g) baby spinach

6-inch (15-cm) length cucumber, peeled and thinly sliced

2 Tbsp avocado oil, coconut oil, or peanut oil

Steamed rice (page 184), for serving (optional)

To make the marinade, in a medium bowl, stir together the soy sauce, miso, fish sauce, garlic, sugar, and pepper. Add the meat and mix to coat all the pieces well. Cover with plastic wrap and marinate at room temperature for about 30 minutes.

Meanwhile, in a small bowl, stir together the vinegar, soy sauce, sugar, and 2 Tbsp water. Add the onions, and set aside. Arrange the spinach and cucumber on a serving plate.

Spread the meat on paper towels and pat dry. In a large frying pan over high heat, heat the oil. When the oil is almost smoking, add half the meat. Let cook without stirring until it is browned and crusty on the bottom, about 2 minutes. Shake the pan vigorously to release the meat, or use tongs to turn the pieces. Cook, shaking the pan to turn the meat until the pieces are well browned on 3 or 4 sides and pink in the center, 5 minutes longer. Arrange the meat on top of the spinach. Add the marinated onions. Serve right away, accompanied with steamed rice, if desired.

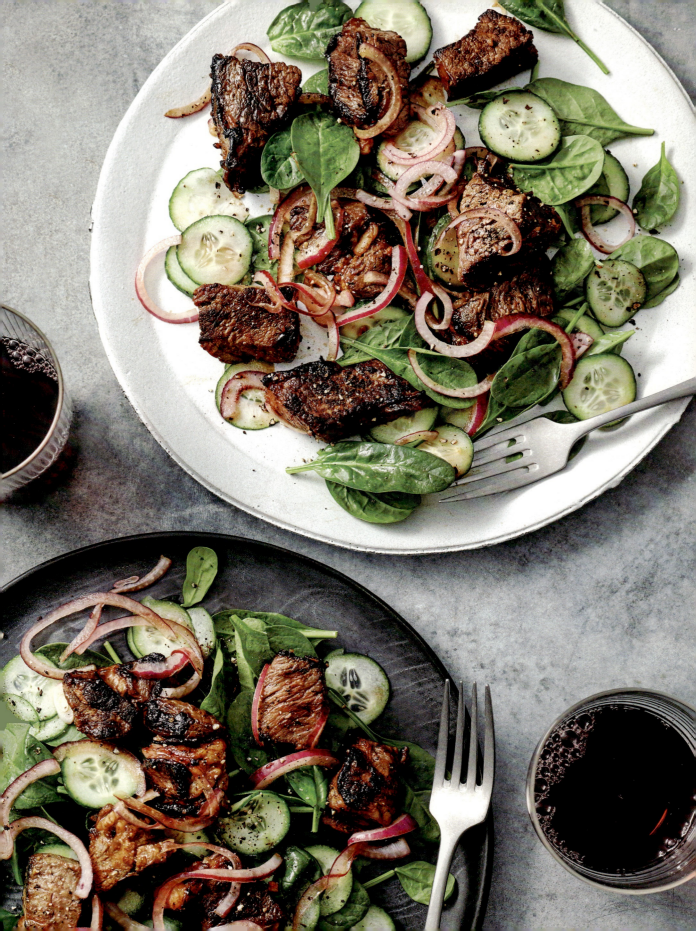

Cider-Braised Pork Tenderloin with Roasted Figs

Figs ripen in mid to late summer, with some varieties producing a second harvest in early fall. They are rich in antioxidants, minerals, and fiber. The best-known fresh figs include Mission, Calimyrna, and Kadota. The sweetness of figs, which roasting accentuates, goes well with roasted meats, a pairing that dates back at least to Roman times.

4 SERVINGS

1 pork tenderloin (about 1 ½ lb/680 g), cut crosswise into 4 medallions

Sea salt and freshly ground black pepper

1 Tbsp olive oil

1 cup (250 ml) hard apple cider

1 sprig fresh rosemary

2 tsp grainy mustard

6 fresh figs, halved lengthwise

1 Tbsp unsalted butter

Preheat the oven to 400°F (200°C). Season the pork with salt and pepper. In an ovenproof frying pan over medium-high heat, heat the olive oil. Brown the pork, turning once, 4–5 minutes total. Transfer to a plate.

Add the cider, rosemary, and mustard to the pan, and bring to a boil, using a wooden spoon to scrape up any browned bits from the pan. Cook until the cider is reduced by half, 3–4 minutes.

Return the pork to the pan, place in the oven, and cook for 6 minutes. Remove from the oven, turn the pork, and add the figs. Return the pan to the oven and cook until the pork is tender and registers 145°F (63°C) on an instant-read thermometer, 6–8 minutes longer. Transfer the pork and figs to a serving platter.

Place the pan over medium heat and whisk in the butter to make a sauce. Spoon the sauce over the top of the pork and figs, and serve right away.

Pork Shoulder with Brussels Sprouts & Tomato Chermoula

Make this slow-roasted dish on Sunday and you'll have lots of flavorful shredded meat, enough high-quality protein for several meals. The pork is roasted simply, using just olive oil, garlic, salt, and pepper. Serve some of it bathed in chermoula, a citrus-sparked North African sauce—you'll still have plenty of leftovers perfect for making tasty tacos and no-fuss hash later in the week.

6 SERVINGS

1 boneless pork shoulder roast (about 4 lb/2 kg) (preferably with a layer of fat intact)

6 Tbsp (90 ml) extra-virgin olive oil

3 cloves garlic, finely chopped

Kosher salt and freshly ground black pepper

1 lb (500 g) Brussels sprouts, trimmed and halved lengthwise

4 Roma (plum) tomatoes, halved lengthwise

¼ cup (7 g) loosely packed fresh cilantro leaves, chopped

¼ cup (7 g) loosely packed fresh flat-leaf parsley leaves, chopped

½ tsp ground cumin

Zest and juice of ½ lemon

Preheat the oven to 425°F (220°C). Line a baking sheet with aluminum foil.

Place the pork shoulder in the center of the prepared pan and coat with 2 Tbsp of the olive oil and the garlic. Season generously with salt and pepper. Roast for 20 minutes, then reduce the oven temperature to 325°F (160°C). Continue roasting until the meat shreds easily and an instant-read thermometer inserted into the center registers 145°F (63°C), about 3 hours longer. Transfer the pork to a cutting board, tent with aluminum foil, and let rest for 30 minutes.

Raise the oven temperature to 500°F (260°C). Line another baking sheet with parchment paper.

In a large bowl, toss together the Brussels sprouts and 2 Tbsp of the olive oil, and season generously with salt and pepper. Place in a single layer on one end of the prepared pan. Brush the tomatoes with 1 Tbsp of the olive oil and season with salt and pepper. Place on the other end of the pan, cut-side down. Roast until the tomatoes begin to char, about 10 minutes. Transfer the tomatoes to a cutting board. Stir the Brussels sprouts and continue roasting until they are fork-tender, about 7 minutes longer. Tent the Brussels sprouts with aluminum foil while you finish the chermoula.

When the tomatoes are cool enough to handle, cut into ½-inch (12-mm) pieces. Transfer to a bowl and stir in the remaining 1 Tbsp olive oil, the cilantro, parsley, cumin, and lemon zest and juice. Season with salt and pepper.

Shred the pork shoulder using 2 forks. Serve with the chermoula and Brussels sprouts on the side.

Lamb Burger with Mint Greek Salad Topping

Here, a lean yet juicy burger is served with mint-scented quinoa in place of a bun—and equally up to absorbing the Greek salad-topped burger's bright flavors. It's a wonderful combination that is gluten-free. Look for sheep's milk feta cheese, which is almost lactose-free and adds a bold taste.

4 SERVINGS

1 cup (180 g) quinoa

Kosher salt and freshly ground black pepper

10 oz (280 g) large Roma (plum) tomatoes, halved and seeded, then finely diced

1 Persian cucumber, finely diced

3 Tbsp diced feta cheese

½ cup (70 g) plus 2 Tbsp finely chopped red onion

½ cup (20 g) fresh mint, chopped

1 ¼ lb (570 g) ground lamb

1 ½ tsp sweet paprika

3 Tbsp extra-virgin olive oil, plus more as needed

Put the quinoa in a fine-mesh strainer. Rinse thoroughly under cold running water and drain. In a saucepan, bring 1 ½ cups (350 ml) water to a boil over high heat. Add the quinoa and a pinch of salt, stir once, and reduce the heat to low. Cover and cook until all the water is absorbed, about 15 minutes. Turn off the heat and let stand for at least 5 minutes.

In a small bowl, mix the tomatoes, cucumber, cheese, 2 Tbsp of the onion, and 2 Tbsp of the mint. Season to taste with salt and pepper.

In another bowl, combine the ground lamb, paprika, remaining ½ cup (70 g) onion, ¼ cup (7 g) of the mint, 1 tsp salt, and a few grindings of pepper; mix gently to blend. Form the lamb mixture into 4 patties, each ½ inch (12 mm) thick. Using your thumb, make an indentation in the center of each patty. Sprinkle with salt and pepper.

In a large frying pan over medium-high heat, heat 2 Tbsp of the olive oil. Add the patties to the pan and cook until done to your liking, about 3 minutes per side for medium-rare.

Fluff the quinoa with a fork. Mix in the remaining 1 Tbsp oil and the remaining 2 Tbsp mint. Season to taste with salt and pepper. Divide the quinoa among serving plates and top each with a lamb patty. Spoon the tomato mixture generously over the patties and quinoa, and serve right away.

TIP *When shaping any burgers, make an indentation with your thumb in the center on one side of the meat patties to help them stay flat during cooking. Without this step, they tend to swell up into a tennis ball shape.*

Five-Spice Pork Tenderloin with Honey-Roasted Edamame

This dish comes together so easily that you may want to roast another tenderloin to use the next day for making sandwiches or serving in warmed flour tortillas with mango salsa (page 187). The honey-roasted edamame—packed with DNA-protecting folate—are so memorable that you won't mind getting your fingers messy.

4 SERVINGS

1 pork tenderloin
(about 1 ¼ lb/570 g)

4 tsp avocado oil, coconut oil,
or peanut oil

2 tsp Chinese five-spice powder

Kosher salt

1 lb (500 g) fresh or thawed
frozen edamame in the shell

2 ½ Tbsp honey

2 Tbsp low-sodium soy sauce

1 clove garlic, minced

¼ tsp red chile flakes (optional)

Preheat the oven to 400°F (200°C). Line a baking sheet with aluminum foil.

Brush the pork tenderloin all over with 2 tsp of the oil and season with the five-spice powder and salt. Place on one end of the prepared pan and roast for 10 minutes.

In a bowl, toss together the edamame, honey, soy sauce, garlic, red chile flakes (if using), and the remaining 2 tsp oil. Pull the pork out of the oven and place the edamame on the other end of the pan. Return the pan to the oven and continue roasting until they are caramelized and an instant-read thermometer inserted into the center of the meat registers 145°F (63°C), 15–20 minutes longer, stirring the edamame halfway through the cooking time.

Transfer the pork to a cutting board, tent with aluminum foil, and let rest for 10 minutes before slicing and serving it with the edamame.

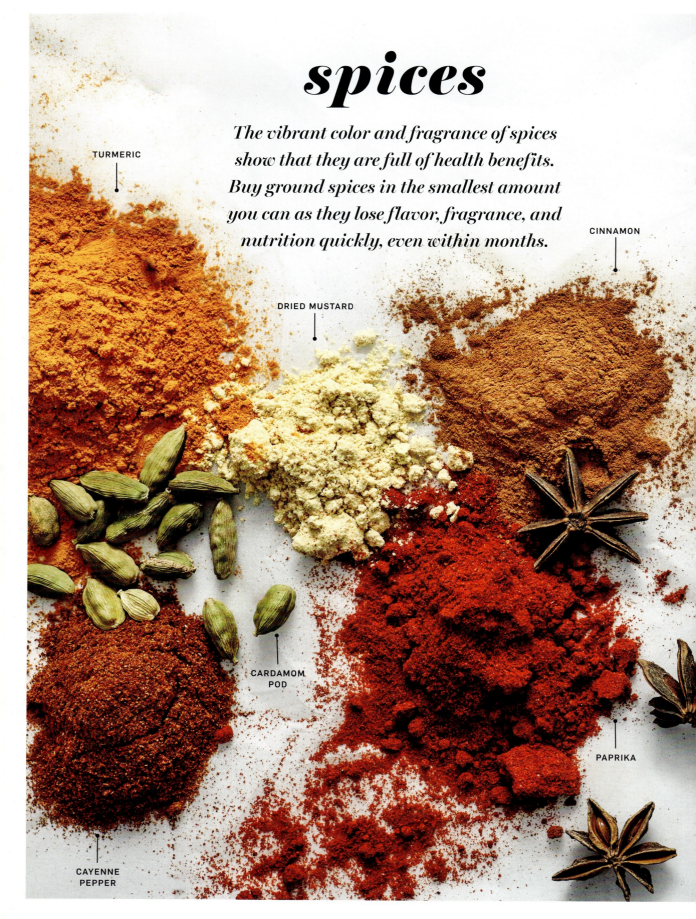

spices

The vibrant color and fragrance of spices show that they are full of health benefits. Buy ground spices in the smallest amount you can as they lose flavor, fragrance, and nutrition quickly, even within months.

TURMERIC

CINNAMON

DRIED MUSTARD

CARDAMOM POD

PAPRIKA

CAYENNE PEPPER

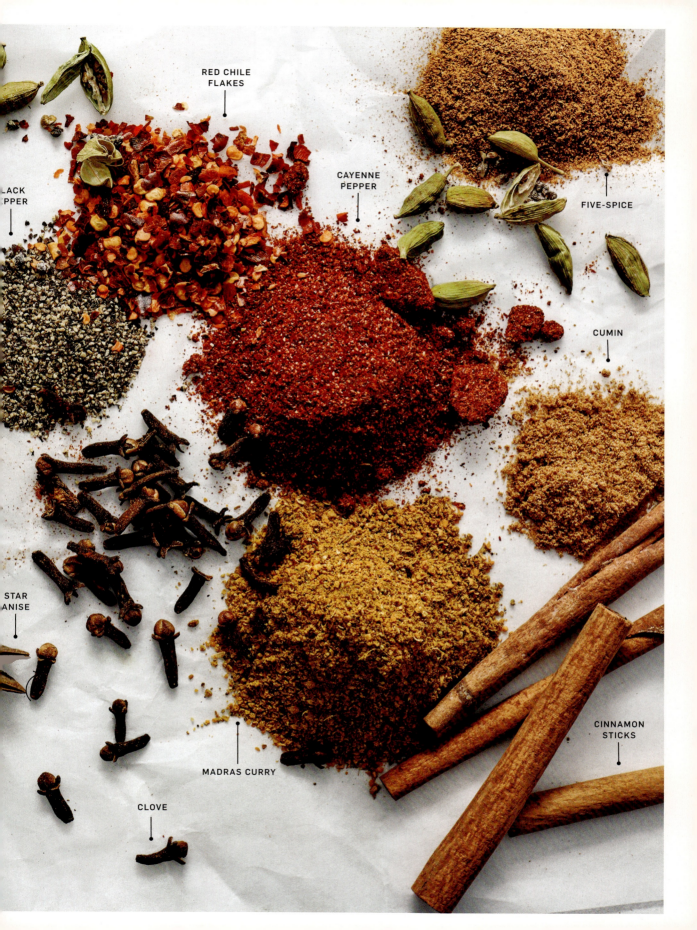

RED CHILE
FLAKES

CAYENNE
PEPPER

FIVE-SPICE

CUMIN

LACK
PPER

STAR
ANISE

MADRAS CURRY

CLOVE

CINNAMON
STICKS

Sweet & Sour Cauliflower with Pan-Seared Tofu

This dish has a secret. Like its Indian-menu inspiration, Manchurian cauliflower, it calls for ketchup. But instead of deep-fried florets, here you'll find roasted cauliflower and the addition of tofu, turning it into a heart-smart main dish. Prepare the rest of dinner while the cauliflower roasts. When the cauliflower and tofu are made ahead, this dish is ready in 15 minutes.

4 SERVINGS

2 lb (1 kg) or 1 small head cauliflower, cut into 1 ½-inch (4-cm) florets

4 Tbsp (60 ml) avocado oil or coconut oil

FOR THE PAN-SEARED TOFU

16–19 oz (500–540 g) firm tofu, drained (see Tips)

Cooking spray

½ cup (60 g) finely chopped red onion

3 cloves garlic, minced

2 tsp peeled and grated fresh ginger

1 ½ tsp garam masala spice blend

1 ½ cups (350 ml) tomato purée

⅓ cup (75 ml) ketchup

⅛–½ tsp ground cayenne pepper (optional)

Preheat the oven to 400°F (200°C). Line a large baking sheet with parchment paper.

Spread the cauliflower on the prepared baking sheet, drizzle with 2 Tbsp of the oil, and toss to coat evenly. Roast until the cauliflower is browned at the edges and crisp-tender, 45 minutes, stirring it once halfway through the cooking time.

To prepare the tofu, cut the block horizontally in half, making two even slabs. Place both pieces on double sheets of paper towel and blot well. Cut each slab into 16 cubes.

Coat a large frying pan liberally with cooking spray and set over medium-high heat. When water flicked into the pan sizzles, add the tofu cubes, placing them ½ inch (12 mm) apart. Cook the cubes until lightly golden on the bottom, 2 minutes. With tongs, turn and cook until the tofu is golden on 3 more sides, 5–6 minutes in all. Set aside. (The seared tofu keeps, tightly covered in the refrigerator, for up to 3 days.)

In a medium nonstick frying pan over medium-high heat, heat the remaining 2 Tbsp oil. When the oil shimmers, add the onion, garlic, and ginger and cook, stirring often, until the onion is golden, 6 minutes. Mix in the garam masala and cook until fragrant, 30 seconds.

Add the tomato purée, ketchup, and cayenne, if using, and mix to combine. Add the roasted cauliflower and seared tofu. Mix to coat them with sauce and cook until heated through, 5 minutes. Serve right away.

TIP *Lightly browning tofu makes it slightly chewy and adds flavor. Sauces cling to the tofu more, as well. Stick with firm tofu. Using a nonstick skillet does not allow the tofu to brown well or develop as much flavor.*

Indian-Spiced Greens with Paneer

This trio of dark greens simmered with pungent ginger, turmeric, garlic, and a touch of coconut is a lean version of classic saag paneer. Don't be alarmed by the immense heap of chopped greens you have—it cooks down to just a few cups. Use the dark, crinkly spinach sometimes called curly or savoy. In place of paneer, vegans can use Pan-Seared Tofu (facing page), or simply omit the cheese.

4 SERVINGS

8 oz (250 g) green chard, stems and center veins removed

8 oz (250 g) mustard greens, stems removed

8 oz (250 g) curly spinach, stems removed

2 Tbsp avocado oil or coconut oil

½ tsp black mustard seeds

1 cup (120 g) finely chopped yellow onion

2 cloves garlic, finely chopped

1 Tbsp peeled and grated fresh ginger

½ tsp ground turmeric

¼–½ tsp red chile flakes (optional)

2 Tbsp unsweetened shredded coconut

½ tsp sea salt

12 oz (350 g) paneer cheese, in ½-inch (12-mm) cubes

Heap the chard, mustard greens, and spinach together and chop them into 2-inch (5-cm) pieces.

In a deep, large frying pan, heat 1 Tbsp of the oil over medium-high heat. Add the mustard seeds and cook, shaking the pan, until they look gray, 2 minutes. Add the onion, garlic, ginger, turmeric, and red chile flakes, if using, and cook, stirring often, until the onion is golden, about 6 minutes.

Add the coconut and half the greens and cook until the greens collapse, 4 minutes. Add the remaining greens in handfuls, stirring occasionally. When the greens have all collapsed and look wet, 10 minutes in total, add the salt and ½ cup (125 ml) water. Spread the greens in an even layer. When the liquid bubbles, reduce the heat and simmer, stirring occasionally, until the greens are slightly chewy, 15–18 minutes. Add just enough water to keep the greens moist, if needed. Transfer the greens to a wide serving bowl.

In the same frying pan, over medium-high heat, warm the remaining 1 Tbsp oil. Add the paneer in one layer, and cook until the cubes are golden on the bottom, 2–3 minutes. With tongs, turn and lightly brown the cheese on 2 more sides, 4 minutes longer. Spoon the cheese over the greens, and serve right away.

Summer Grilled Pizza

This pizza looks best topped with a combination of cherry, grape, or other small tomatoes in any combination of colors. Since the skin holds most of a tomato's lycopene and other antioxidants, using smaller tomatoes provides more skin per serving—and delivers more of these healthful phytonutrients. But you can thinly slice two large tomatoes instead, remove the seeds and gently blot any excess moisure to prevent a soggy pizza.

1 LARGE PIZZA

1 ½ cups (340 g) cherry tomatoes, stemmed and halved

2 Tbsp olive oil, plus more for brushing

2 cloves garlic, pressed

Kosher salt

Unbleached all-purpose flour, for dusting

About ¾ lb (350 g) pizza dough (page 189)

1 ¼ cups (5 oz/140 g) shredded whole-milk mozzarella cheese

1 cup (4 oz/120 g) crumbled Gorgonzola cheese

2 green onions, thinly sliced

2 Tbsp chopped fresh basil leaves

1 Tbsp chopped fresh marjoram or oregano leaves

(V) (SF)

In a bowl, combine the tomatoes, 1 Tbsp of the olive oil, and 1 garlic clove. Sprinkle with salt and stir to blend. In a small bowl, mix the remaining garlic clove with the remaining 1 Tbsp olive oil.

Prepare a charcoal or gas grill for direct-heat cooking over medium heat. Meanwhile, on a lightly floured work surface, roll out the dough into a rectangle about 11 x 13 inches (28 x 33 cm). Brush the top surface of the dough with olive oil.

Place the dough on the grill, oiled-side down, and immediately brush the top of the crust with the garlic oil. Grill until well browned on the bottom, about 5 minutes. Using a wide spatula, carefully turn the pizza crust over, and immediately sprinkle with the mozzarella and Gorgonzola cheeses. Distribute the tomato mixture evenly over the cheeses, and sprinkle evenly with the green onions, basil, and marjoram. Grill until the pizza is just browned on the bottom and the cheeses melt, 6–8 minutes.

Using the spatula or a rimless baking sheet, transfer the pizza to a cutting board. Cut the pizza into squares, and serve right away.

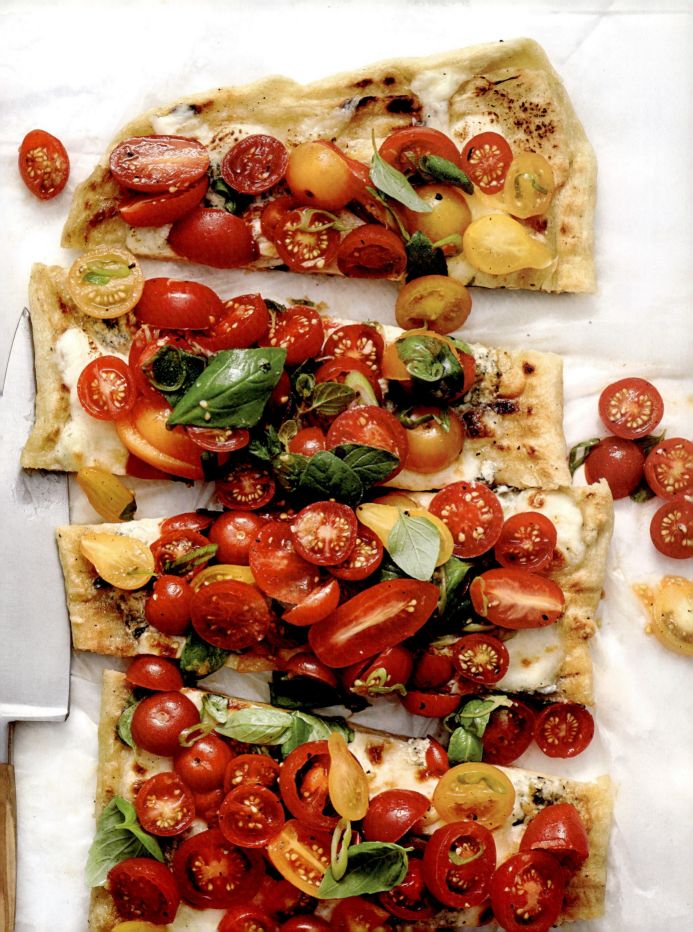

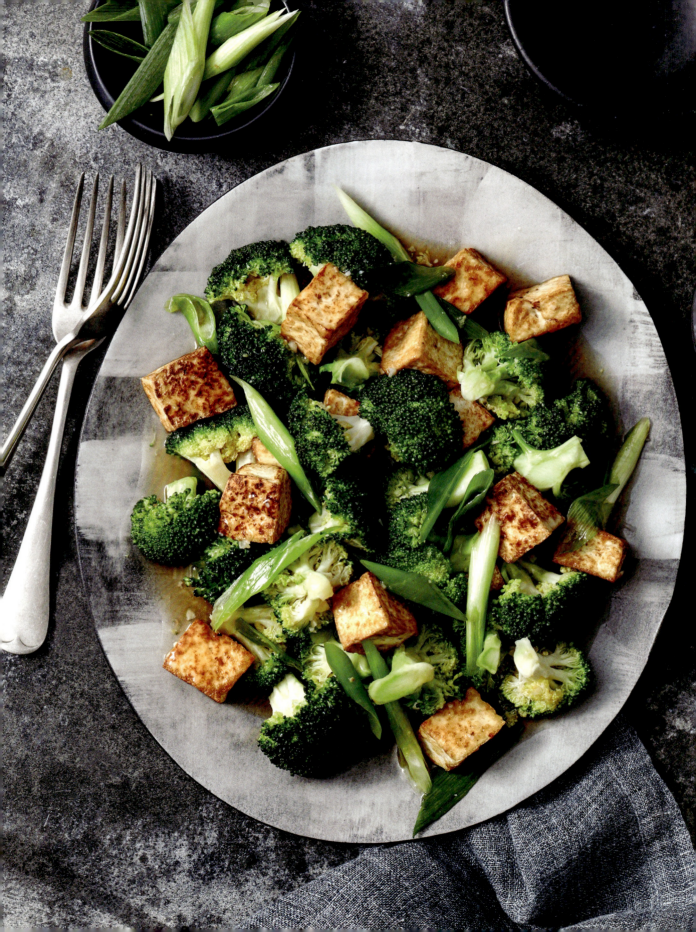

General Tso's Tofu with Broccoli

This vegetarian version delivers the same sweet heat people love in the original. Pan-seared tofu is remarkably close in texture to the fried chicken it replaces while broccoli brings cruciferous goodness. Leftovers served at room temperature are tasty the next day. To make this dish gluten-free, replace the soy sauce with tamari.

4 SERVINGS

FOR THE PAN-SEARED TOFU

16–19 oz (500–540 g) firm tofu, drained (see Tips)

Cooking spray

FOR THE SAUCE

¾ cup (180 ml) vegetable broth

2 Tbsp maple syrup

1 Tbsp low-sodium soy sauce

1 tsp Sriracha or other hot chile sauce

2 tsp cornstarch

2 Tbsp peanut oil, avocado oil, or coconut oil

⅓ cup (30 g) chopped green onions, white and green parts

2 cloves garlic, finely chopped

1 Tbsp peeled and grated fresh ginger

4 cups (12 oz/350 g) bite-size broccoli florets

2 tsp sesame oil

To prepare the tofu, cut the block horizontally in half, making two even slabs. Place both pieces on double sheets of paper towel and blot well. Cut each slab into 16 cubes.

Coat a large frying pan liberally with oil spray and set over medium-high heat. When water flicked into the pan sizzles, add the tofu cubes, placing them ½ inch (12 mm) apart. Cook the cubes until lightly golden on the bottom, 2 minutes. With tongs, turn and cook until the tofu is golden on 3 more sides, 5–6 minutes in all. Set aside. (The seared tofu keeps, tightly covered in the refrigerator, for up to 3 days.)

To make the sauce, in a small bowl, stir together ½ cup (125 ml) of the broth, the maple syrup, soy sauce, Sriracha, and cornstarch. Set aside.

In a wok or large nonstick frying pan over high heat, heat the oil. When the oil is shimmering, add the green onions, garlic, and ginger and stir-fry with a wooden spatula until they are fragrant, 30 seconds. Add the broccoli and stir-fry until it is bright green, 1 minute. Add the remaining ¼ cup (60 ml) broth and cook, stirring, until the broccoli is tender-crisp, about 2 minutes.

Give the sauce a quick stir. Add the tofu, sauce, and sesame oil to the pan and stir until the sauce thickens, about 1 minute. Serve right away.

TIP *Lightly browning tofu gives it nutty flavor and makes it slightly chewy. This makes it more appealing when added to dishes. Sauces cling to the tofu more, as well. Stick with firm tofu. Avoid using a nonstick skillet, which does not allow the tofu to develop as much flavor.*

Mexican Quinoa & Vegetable Casserole

This protein-packed dish is reminiscent of an old-school taco casserole, but instead of ground beef and rice, here you'll find seitan (wheat gluten) and red quinoa. The result is a quick and filling meal that satisfies Mexican food cravings in a new, healthy way.

4 SERVINGS

¾ cup (135 g) red quinoa, drained and rinsed

Sea salt and freshly ground black pepper

2 Tbsp olive oil

1 cup (140 g) finely chopped yellow onion

1 small red bell pepper, seeded and chopped

1 cup (180 g) frozen corn kernels

½ lb (250 g) seitan (wheat gluten), chopped or crumbled

1 Tbsp chili powder

1 can (15 oz/425 g) black beans, drained and rinsed

½ cup (125 ml) jarred tomato salsa

1 cup (4 oz/120 g) shredded pepper Jack cheese

½ cup (20 g) chopped fresh cilantro (optional)

In a small saucepan, bring 1 ¼ cups (300 ml) water to a boil over high heat. Add the quinoa and ½ tsp salt, reduce the heat to medium-low, cover, and cook until tender, about 15 minutes.

In a large ovenproof frying pan over medium-high heat, heat the olive oil. Add the onion, bell pepper, corn, seitan, and chili powder and cook until the vegetables are tender, about 5 minutes. Reduce the heat to low and fold in the beans and salsa; cook for 1 minute. Remove the pan from the heat and gently fold in the quinoa. Season to taste with salt and pepper.

Place a rack in the top third of the oven and preheat the broiler. Sprinkle the quinoa mixture evenly with the cheese. Broil until the cheese is melted and bubbly, about 5 minutes. Sprinkle with the cilantro, if using, and serve.

TIP *Save a step and buy a packet of precooked quinoa, available in shelf-stable bags and in the freezer department of grocery stores. You will need about 2 cups (370 g) cooked quinoa for this recipe.*

Braised Chickpeas & Carrots with Yogurt

In this easy weeknight dish, tender beans and sweet carrots are infused with enticing spices, and get a dollop of an Indian-inspired yogurt topping. White quinoa is a great substitute for couscous, if you are avoiding gluten, and it is very high in protein.

4 SERVINGS

1 lb (500 g) slender carrots, unpeeled

4 Tbsp (60 ml) plus 1 ½ tsp olive oil

1 large yellow onion, coarsely chopped

2 tsp sweet paprika

1 tsp ground cumin

½ tsp ground cinnamon

½ tsp ground ginger

¼ tsp cayenne pepper

2 cans (15 oz/425 g each) chickpeas, drained and rinsed

2 cans (14.5 oz/411 g each) diced tomatoes with juices

1 cup (150 g) raisins

Kosher salt and freshly ground black pepper

1 ½ cups (270 g) quinoa

½ cup (125 g) plain Greek-style yogurt

Fresh cilantro leaves and toasted sliced almonds, for garnish

Halve the carrots lengthwise and then quarter them crosswise. In a large nonstick frying pan over medium heat, heat 2 Tbsp of the oil. Add the onion and carrots and sauté until the onion is tender, about 5 minutes. Add the paprika, cumin, cinnamon, ginger, and cayenne and stir for 10 seconds. Add the chickpeas, tomatoes with juices, raisins, and 1 cup (250 ml) water. Sprinkle with salt and pepper. Bring to a boil over high heat, reduce the heat to medium-low, cover, and simmer until the carrots are just tender, about 20 minutes.

Put the quinoa in a fine-mesh strainer. Rinse thoroughly under cold running water and drain. In a saucepan, bring 2 ¼ cups (530 ml) water to a boil over high heat. Add the quinoa and a pinch of salt, stir once, and reduce the heat to low. Cover and cook, without stirring, until all the water is absorbed and the grains are tender, about 15 minutes. Turn off the heat and let stand for at least 5 minutes.

In a small bowl, mix the yogurt and 1 Tbsp of the olive oil. Season to taste with salt and pepper. Fluff the quinoa with a fork, and then mix in the remaining 1 Tbsp plus 1 ½ tsp olive oil.

Divide the quinoa among serving plates. Season the chickpea mixture to taste with salt and pepper and spoon it over the quinoa. Spoon the yogurt on top. Sprinkle with cilantro and almonds, and serve.

TIP *For the topping, choose the yogurt you like best—whole milk, two percent, fat free, or nondairy. No side dish is needed for this complete dish.*

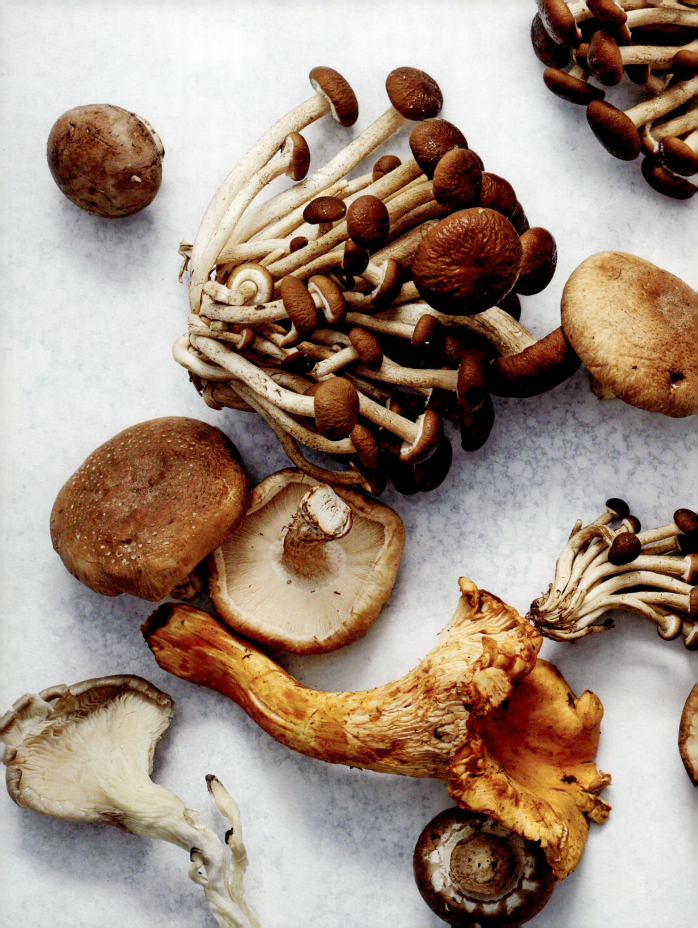

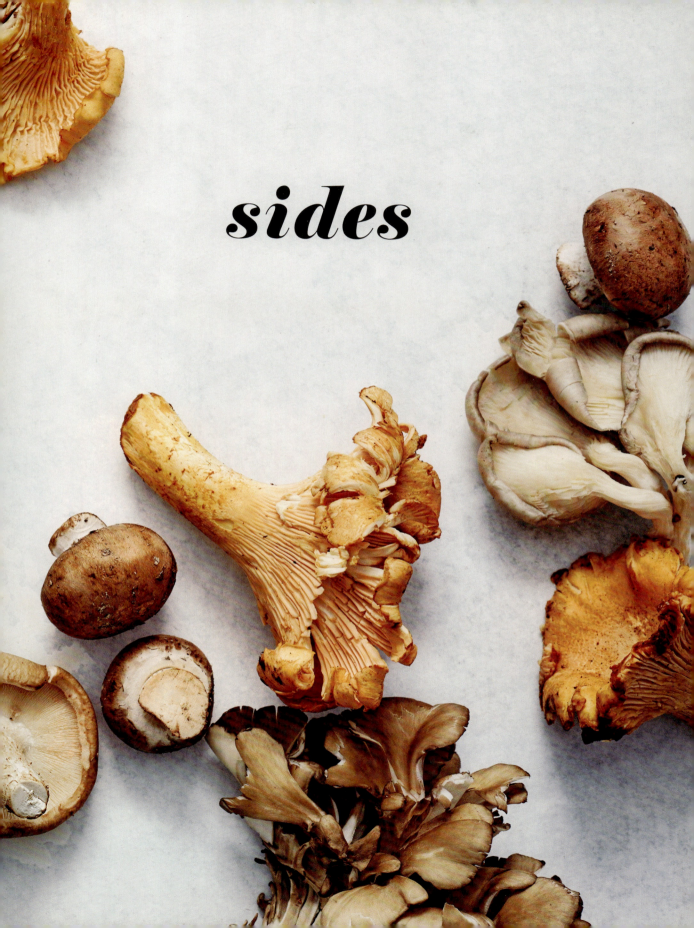

sides

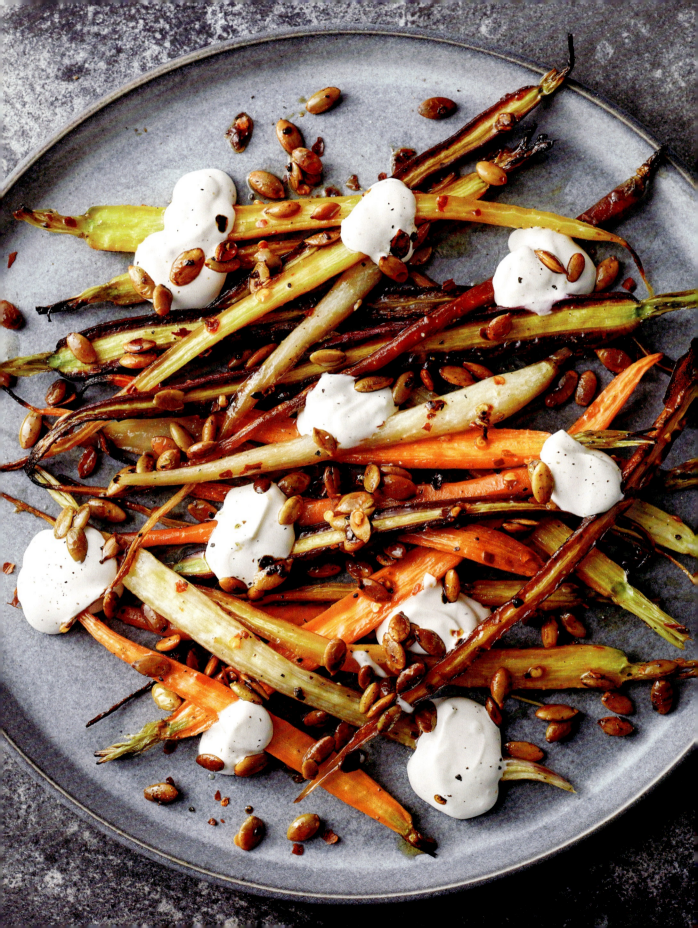

Chile-Honey Roasted Carrots

The carrots and yogurt play beautifully in this dish, with the roasted carrots'
spicy sweetness cut by the creamy tang of the yogurt. It goes well with protein-
heavy chicken or pork main dishes. For a satisfying vegetarian meal, pair this
with Cauliflower Steaks with Olive-Caper Gremolata (page 139).

4 SERVINGS

1 lb (500 g) rainbow carrots, trimmed, peeled, and halved lengthwise if large

¼ cup (60 ml) extra-virgin olive oil

2 Tbsp honey

Kosher salt and freshly ground black pepper

2 tsp red chile flakes

FOR THE YOGURT TOPPING

½ cup (125 g) plain whole-milk Greek yogurt

1 Tbsp extra-virgin olive oil

Kosher salt and freshly ground black pepper

FOR THE SEASONED PUMPKIN SEEDS

3 Tbsp extra-virgin olive oil

⅓ cup (50 g) raw pumpkin seeds

Kosher salt and freshly ground black pepper

½ tsp sweet paprika

½ tsp red chile flakes

Flaky sea salt, for finishing

Preheat the oven to 375°F (190°C). Pile the carrots on a baking sheet. In a small bowl, whisk together the olive oil and honey. Drizzle the oil mixture over the carrots and toss the carrots to coat evenly. Season with salt and pepper, then sprinkle with the red chile flakes and toss again. Arrange the carrots in a single layer and roast until tender, 25–30 minutes.

Meanwhile, make the yogurt topping and seasoned pumpkin seeds. To make the topping, in a small bowl, whisk together the yogurt and olive oil, mixing well. Season to taste with salt and pepper. Set aside.

To make the seasoned pumpkin seeds, in a small frying pan over medium heat, heat the olive oil. Add the pumpkin seeds, a pinch each of salt and pepper, the paprika, and the red chile flakes and toast, stirring frequently, until the seeds are fragrant and lightly golden, 3–5 minutes. Remove from the heat and season to taste with salt and pepper.

Transfer the carrots to a serving platter. Top with small dollops of the yogurt topping and with the pumpkin seeds. Sprinkle with flaky sea salt. Serve warm or at room temperature.

Roasted Beets with Indian Spices

A quartet of spices commonly used in Indian-style curry blends works magic on simple roasted beets. During cooking, the spice mixture penetrates the beets, flavoring them even after they are peeled. Beets are rich in nitrates that help lower blood pressure, making them a good vegetable to eat regularly.

4 SERVINGS

1 tsp ground cumin

1 tsp ground coriander

½ tsp ground turmeric

½ tsp ground cloves

Kosher salt and freshly ground black pepper

6 beets (about 30 oz/850 g total weight), stems trimmed to ½ inch (12 mm)

2 Tbsp extra-virgin olive oil, plus more as needed

Flaky sea salt, for finishing

Preheat the oven to 350°F (180°C). In a small bowl, combine the cumin, coriander, turmeric, and cloves with 1 tsp salt and 1 tsp pepper. Stir to mix.

Arrange the beets in a shallow roasting pan just large enough to hold them in a single layer. Drizzle them with the olive oil, then sprinkle with the spice mixture, turning to coat. Roast, turning occasionally, until the skins are slightly wrinkled and the beets are tender when pierced with a knife, about 1 ¼ hours.

When the beets are cool enough to handle, cut off the stems and peel them. Cut the beets lengthwise into wedges, drizzle with additional olive oil if desired, and sprinkle with flaky sea salt and pepper. Serve right away, warm or at room temperature.

Spicy Roasted Broccoli with Garlic

This minimalist dish takes advantage of the entire stalk of broccoli—even the usually discarded stems, which contain the same detoxifying compounds useful in cancer prevention as the florets. You can also make this recipe with broccolini, broccoli's smaller, sweeter, more tender cousin, though it does provide fewer vitamins and minerals overall.

4–6 SERVINGS

1 ½ lb (680 g) broccoli heads, trimmed

¼ cup (60 ml) olive oil

3 Tbsp fresh lemon juice, plus more for serving

3 cloves garlic, minced

Pinch of red chile flakes

Sea salt

Preheat the oven to 400°F (200°C). Cut the broccoli lengthwise into spears 4–6 inches (10–15 cm) long. Using a vegetable peeler or a sharp paring knife, remove any dried or bruised skin from the stems. Arrange the spears in a single layer in a roasting pan. Drizzle with the oil, then sprinkle with the lemon juice, garlic, salt, and red chile flakes. Toss to coat.

Roast until the broccoli is tender and the tips and outer edges are crisp and browned, about 15 minutes, turning the spears once about halfway through cooking. Serve right away with an extra squeeze of lemon juice and salt to taste.

Baby Bok Choy, Shiitake Mushroom & Sugar Snap Pea Stir-Fry

Stir-frying quickly over high heat lets vegetables keep more of their valuable micronutrients. It also lets you prepare this flavorful dish in minutes. Cutting the mushrooms by hand into generous strips enhances their presence. Peanut oil is traditional for stir-fries and takes heat well, but using other oils with a high smoke point, like avocado oil or coconut oil, is fine.

4 SERVINGS

¼ cup (60 ml) low-sodium vegetable broth

1 Tbsp low-sodium soy sauce

2 tsp rice vinegar

½ tsp sugar

1 tsp cornstarch

1 Tbsp peanut oil, avocado oil, or coconut oil

4 cloves garlic, smashed and peeled

1-inch (2.5-cm) piece fresh ginger, peeled, sliced, and thinly shredded

2 cups (180 g) fresh shiitake mushrooms, sliced ½ inch (12 mm) thick

2 cups (200 g) sugar snap peas

12 oz (350 g) baby bok choy, halved or quartered lengthwise

2 tsp toasted sesame oil

In a small bowl, stir together the broth, soy sauce, vinegar, sugar, and cornstarch to make a sauce. Set aside.

In a large frying pan over medium-high heat, heat the oil. When the oil is shimmering, add the garlic and ginger and stir-fry with a wooden spatula until they are fragrant, about 30 seconds. Add the mushrooms and stir-fry until they squeak, about 1 minute. Add the sugar snap peas and bok choy and use tongs to turn and stir them until they are bright green, about 2 minutes.

Give the sauce a quick stir and add it to the pan. Stir-fry until it thickens and coats the vegetables, about 1 minute. Sprinkle on the sesame oil, stir, and serve right away.

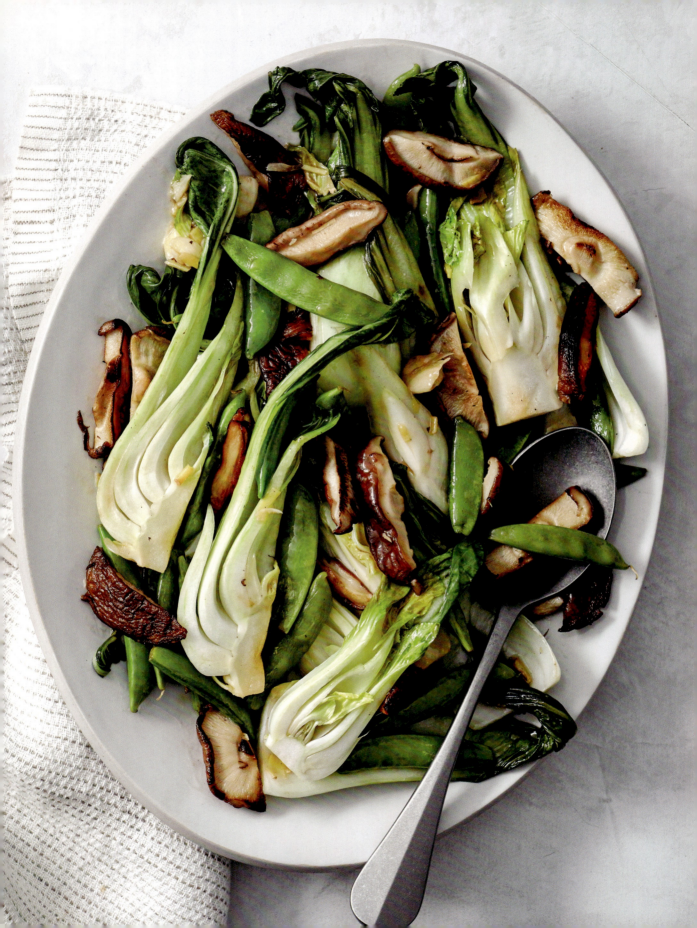

Oven-Roasted Tomatoes with Herbs

Roasting intensifies the flavor of tomatoes, and these are fantastic served alongside roast meats, sautéed fish, or as a condiment on sandwiches. They are an ideal way to add micronutrients to a protein-centered meal. Chilled, drizzled with olive oil and balsamic vinegar, they make an elegant starter. You can also purée them to use as a zesty sauce on pizza or pasta.

6 SERVINGS

2 Tbsp olive oil, plus more for greasing

2 lb (1 kg) small round Roma (plum) tomatoes, halved through the stem end

2 cloves garlic, pressed

1 Tbsp minced fresh oregano leaves

2 tsp minced fresh thyme leaves

¼ tsp kosher salt

Preheat the oven to 375°F (190°C). Grease a large, heavy rimmed baking sheet with olive oil.

In a bowl, toss together the tomatoes, the 2 Tbsp olive oil, garlic, oregano, and thyme. Arrange the tomatoes, cut sides up, on the prepared baking sheet. Sprinkle the tomatoes with the salt. Roast the tomatoes until they are soft and beginning to brown, about 50 minutes. Let the tomatoes cool to room temperature on the baking sheet. Serve at room temperature or chilled.

Smashed Potatoes with Paprika Salt

Though carbs have gotten flak in recent years, they should typically make up 45 to 65 percent of a healthy diet as they are a long-lasting source of energy for both your brain and muscles. Smashing rather than mashing these lower-starch red and yellow potatoes turns the insides creamy while the skins stay crackly. If you don't have smoked paprika, add additional sweet paprika plus dashes of cumin and coriander.

4 SERVINGS

2 lb (1 kg) small red or Yukon Gold potatoes

Sea salt

1 tsp sweet paprika

½ tsp smoked paprika

3 Tbsp extra-virgin olive oil

Preheat the oven to 400°F (200°C). Line a rimmed baking sheet with parchment paper. In a large saucepan, combine the potatoes with water to cover by 2 inches (5 cm). Salt the water generously, bring to a boil over high heat, and cook, uncovered, until the potatoes are just tender when pierced with a knife, 12–15 minutes.

While the potatoes are cooking, in a small bowl, stir together 1 tsp sea salt, the sweet paprika, and the smoked paprika.

Drain the potatoes in a colander and transfer them to a bowl. Drizzle with 2 Tbsp of the olive oil, sprinkle with the paprika salt, and toss until the potatoes are evenly coated. Spread the potatoes in a single layer on the prepared baking sheet. Using the heel of your hand or the back of a wooden spoon, smash each potato until it splits and flattens slightly. Pour the remaining 1 Tbsp olive oil into the bowl used to season the potatoes and stir to mix it with the spices left in the bowl. Brush the mixture over the tops of the smashed potatoes.

Roast the potatoes until the skins are crisp, about 35 minutes. Serve right away.

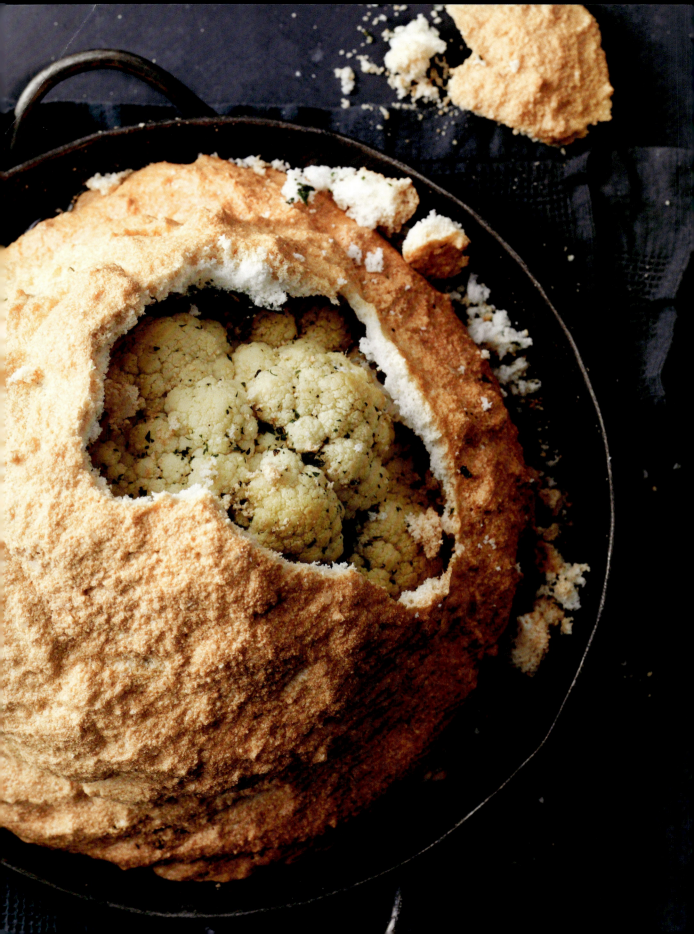

Salt-Crusted Whole Cauliflower

Cauliflower's recent ascension to vegetable superstardom is due in part to its low carb content, high nutritional value, and versatility. From pizza crust to steak substitute, its appeal comes from its ability to showcase surrounding flavors without competing. Here, it highlights an aromatic herbal medley of fresh sage, parsley, and thyme. Feel free to swap in herbs and spices to your liking.

4–6 SERVINGS

1 head cauliflower
(about 2 lb/1 kg)

4 large egg whites

2 cups (270 g) kosher salt

1 Tbsp chopped fresh sage

1 Tbsp chopped fresh flat-leaf parsley

1 tsp fresh thyme leaves

3 Tbsp olive oil

Green onion tops, thinly sliced, for garnish

Sesame seeds, for garnish

Preheat the oven to 425°F (220°C). Remove the leaves and tough core of the cauliflower, keeping the head intact.

In a stand mixer fitted with the whisk attachment, or in a large bowl using a handheld mixer, beat the egg whites on high speed until soft peaks form when the whisk is lifted, about 3 minutes. Using a rubber spatula, gently fold in the salt until a wet foam forms.

In a small bowl, stir together the sage, parsley, thyme, and olive oil, mixing well. Rub the oil mixture evenly over the cauliflower, including the underside. In a cast-iron frying pan, spread some of the egg white mixture into a round ½ inch (12 mm) thick large enough to fit the cauliflower. Set the cauliflower on the circle, stem-side down, then spread the remaining egg white mixture evenly over the entire surface of the cauliflower. Use your fingertips to pat the mixture in place, making sure there are no gaps.

Roast until the egg white crust is hardened and golden brown and the cauliflower is tender when pierced with a knife, about 45 minutes. Let cool for 5 minutes, then crack the crust with a knife and remove and discard the crust. Cut the cauliflower into wedges and serve.

Carrot Noodles with Kale Pesto

Cook this pasta stand-in until nicely al dente, then toss it with bold kale pesto for a colorful, superfoody side dish. Add pan-seared tofu (page 119) or shredded rotisserie chicken to make it a complete one-dish meal, if you like. Leftover carrot noodles are a good addition to salad.

4 SERVINGS

2 Tbsp olive oil

16 oz (500 g) carrot noodles (see Tip)

½ cup (120 ml) Kale Pesto (page 186)

½ cup (2 oz/60 g) grated Parmesan cheese

In large frying pan over medium-high heat, heat the olive oil. Add the carrot noodles. Using tongs, stir and turn to coat the carrots with the oil. Continue to stir and turn the carrots every 30 seconds until they are crisp-tender, about 5 minutes. Add the pesto and stir until the carrots are evenly coated.

Transfer the cooked noodles to a serving bowl. Top with the cheese, and serve right away.

TIP *Use a spiralizer or julienne peeler to make carrot noodles, or look for them in the bagged salad section of the supermarket.*

Braised Moroccan Eggplant

Similar to, though smaller than, the American globe eggplant, the Italian variety is deep purple, oblong, and wider at the blossom end than the stem end. An antioxidant found in its purple skin has been shown in studies to protect our skin and brain cell membranes from damage caused by free radicals. Salting the eggplant keeps this versatile vegetable from absorbing too much oil by drawing moisture from the plant cells into air pockets in its flesh.

4 SERVINGS

1 large Italian eggplant (about 1 lb/500 g), trimmed and cut into ½-inch (12-mm) cubes

Kosher salt

1 tsp ground cumin

1 tsp sweet paprika

½ tsp ground coriander

1 can (14 oz/400 g) whole Roma (plum) tomatoes, with juice

¼ cup (60 ml) olive oil

2 cloves garlic, smashed

½ cup (30 g) chopped fresh mint

½ cup (30 g) chopped fresh cilantro

2 Tbsp minced preserved lemon peel (optional)

Put the eggplant cubes in a colander, sprinkle with 2 tsp salt, and toss to coat evenly. Set the colander in a sink and let the eggplant stand for 10 minutes (liquid will bead up on the flesh).

Meanwhile, in a small bowl, stir together the cumin, paprika, and coriander. Pour the tomatoes and their juice into a bowl and crush the tomatoes with your hand or a potato masher.

In a large sauté pan or wok over medium-high heat, heat the olive oil and garlic. Swirl the pan to flavor the oil with the garlic until the garlic starts to sizzle but does not color, about 1 minute. Add the eggplant (do not rinse off the salt) and stir until well coated with the oil. Pour in ¼ cup (60 ml) water and bring it to a boil. Cover, reduce the heat to medium-low, and cook until the eggplant is tender, about 10 minutes. Uncover and gently stir in the tomatoes. Raise the heat to medium-high and let cook, uncovered, at a brisk simmer, shaking the pan occasionally, until the tomatoes thicken into a sauce, about 10 minutes longer.

Remove from the heat, gently stir in the mint and cilantro, and remove and discard the garlic, if desired. Transfer the eggplant to a serving dish, sprinkle with the preserved lemon, if using, and serve warm or at room temperature.

Edamame, Corn & Sweet Onion Succotash

Early Native Americans created succotash by combining maize and any kind of beans to make a stew. Here, edamame and corn come together in a comforting side dish with enough protein from the nutty, sweet-tasting soybeans to anchor a light meal. It keeps well and tastes good at room temperature, so take leftover succotash for lunch the next day.

4 SERVINGS

Sea salt and freshly ground black pepper

4 oz (120 g) frozen shelled edamame (1 cup)

8 oz (250 g) frozen or fresh yellow corn kernels (about 2 cups)

½ cup (60 g) finely chopped red onion

½ cup (125 ml) low-sodium chicken or vegetable broth

Pinch of cayenne pepper

2 Tbsp butter

Bring a medium saucepan of well-salted water to a boil. Add the edamame and cook for 5 minutes. Drain and return the edamame to the pan.

Add the corn, onion, broth, and cayenne to the edamame. Bring the liquid to a boil over medium-high heat, reduce the heat, cover, and simmer until the corn is crisp-tender, 3 minutes. Off the heat, mix in the butter. Season with salt and pepper to taste. Serve right away.

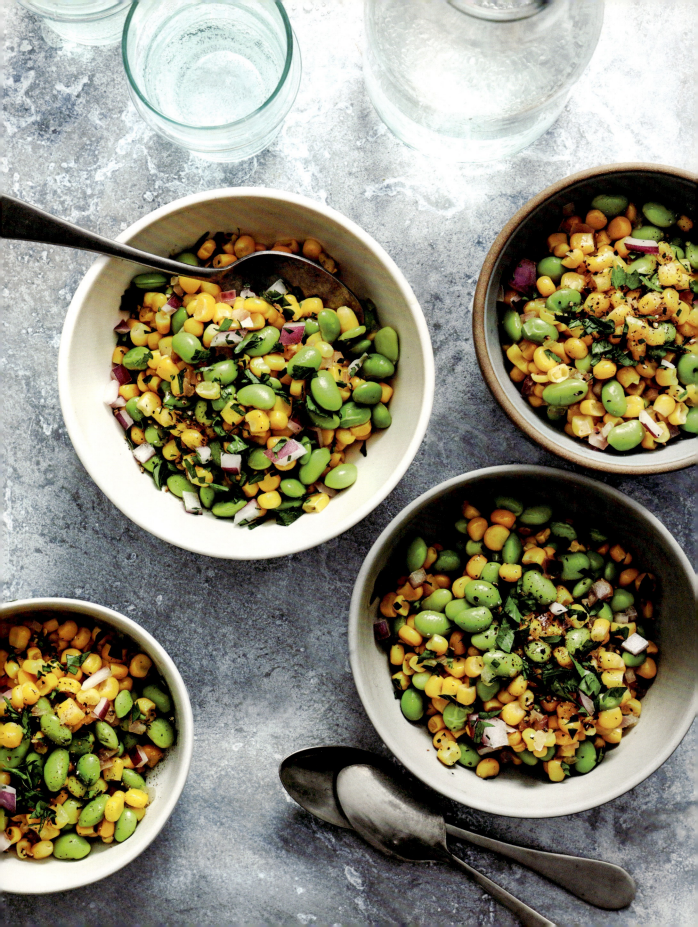

Braised Lacinato Kale with Apples & Carrots

Carrots and apples offer natural sweetness that contrasts nicely with kale's muscular taste. Kale and red cabbage are packed with the detoxifying compounds found in all crucifers. Red cabbage gets its color from anthocyanins, pigments that are also protective antioxidants. Cider and ginger add bright flavors you'll find welcome in fall and winter.

4 SERVINGS

1 Tbsp coconut oil or avocado oil

4 oz (120 g) shredded red cabbage (2 cups)

½ cup (60 g) chopped red onion

12 oz (350 g) lacinato kale, cut into ½-inch (12-mm) strips (about 6 cups)

¾ cup (90 g) coarsely shredded carrots

1 small Fuji apple, cored and thinly sliced

1 tsp peeled and grated fresh ginger

½ cup (125 ml) apple cider

1 Tbsp apple cider vinegar

Sea salt and freshly ground black pepper

VG V GF DF SF

In a large frying pan over medium-high heat, heat the oil. When the oil is shimmering, add the cabbage and onion and cook, stirring a few times, until coated with oil and tender, about 4 minutes.

Mix in the kale and cook, stirring occasionally. When the kale looks slick, about 4 minutes, add the carrots, apple, ginger, cider, and vinegar. When the liquid begins to bubble, reduce the heat and simmer gently until the kale is crisp-tender, about 10 minutes. Season with salt and pepper. Serve right away.

Seared Cauliflower Steaks with Olive-Caper Gremolata

Well-seasoned cauliflower steaks can be a satisfying swap for red meat. Cutting more than two steaks from a head of cauliflower is difficult because each slice needs to include a good section of the core to hold it together. This leaves a pile of smaller florets ideal for adding to another dish. Try Moroccan Roast Chicken & Vegetables (page 96) or Sweet & Sour Cauliflower with Pan-Seared Tofu (page 114).

4 SERVINGS

FOR THE GREMOLATA

1 rib celery, finely chopped

1 green onion, white and pale green parts, finely chopped

2 Tbsp salted capers, rinsed and finely chopped

4 large green olives, preferably Bella di Cerignola, pitted and finely chopped

1 ½ Tbsp chopped fresh dill

Grated zest of 1 orange

2 small heads white, green, or orange cauliflower

4 Tbsp olive oil

2 cloves garlic, smashed

⅛–¼ tsp red chile flakes

Sea salt and freshly ground black pepper

To make the gremolata, in a bowl, stir together the celery, green onion, capers, olives, dill, and orange zest. Set aside.

Trim the base of 1 head of cauliflower, removing all the greens but keeping as much of the stem as possible intact. Using a large serrated knife, carefully slice the cauliflower through the middle of the stem to create 2 halves, then cut off the rounded outer parts of each half to create a total of 2 steaks, each about 1 ¼ inches (3 cm) thick and flat on both sides; reserve the crumbly outer florets for another use. Repeat with the second head of cauliflower.

In each of 2 large frying pans (preferably cast iron), warm 2 Tbsp of the olive oil over medium-low heat. Divide the garlic and red chile flakes between the pans, and season generously with salt and pepper. Add 2 cauliflower steaks to each pan and cook without moving until golden brown, 4–5 minutes; maintain a low sizzle so the cauliflower doesn't scorch. Using a wide spatula, turn the steaks over and cook on the second sides until golden brown, 4–5 minutes longer. Remove the pans from the heat, cover, and let the cauliflower steaks steam for 5 minutes to help them soften; they should be tender when pierced with a skewer.

Transfer the cauliflower steaks to a serving platter, scatter with a generous amount of the gremolata, and serve right away.

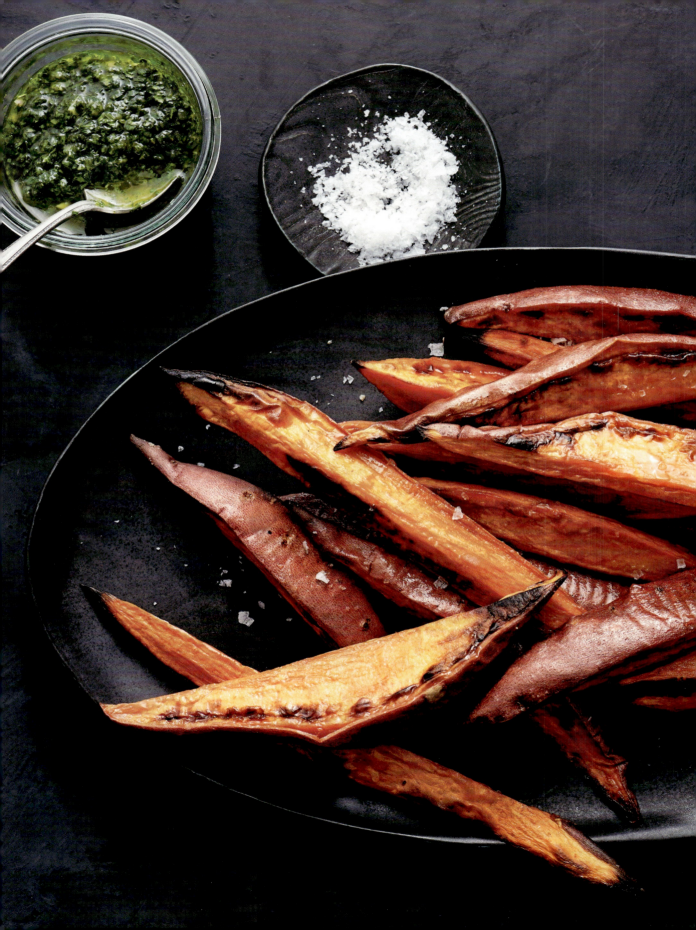

Baked Sweet Potatoes
with Chile-Lime Butter

With some vegetables, bigger does not mean better. For the best flavor, look for small sweet potatoes at your greengrocer of farmers' market. Make sure the butter is quite soft before mixing in the lime juice so that the juice gets fully incorporated. If you limit unsaturated fats, swap the butter for an extra-virgin or basil-infused olive oil.

4 SERVINGS

4 orange-fleshed sweet potatoes (about 6 oz/180 g each)

4 Tbsp (60 g) unsalted butter, at room temperature

1 Tbsp ancho chile powder

1 Tbsp fresh lime juice

1 tsp honey

¼ tsp grated lime zest

¼ tsp kosher salt

Preheat the oven to 425°F (220°C). Pierce the unpeeled sweet potatoes in a few spots with a small, sharp knife and place on a rimmed baking sheet. Bake until tender when pierced with a fork, about 50 minutes.

While the sweet potatoes are baking, in a small bowl, stir together the butter, chile powder, lime juice, honey, lime zest, and salt until well blended.

When the sweet potatoes are ready, remove from the oven, slit each sweet potato lengthwise down the center to open, then place on a platter or serving dish. Top the sweet potatoes with the flavored butter, or serve alongside, and serve right away.

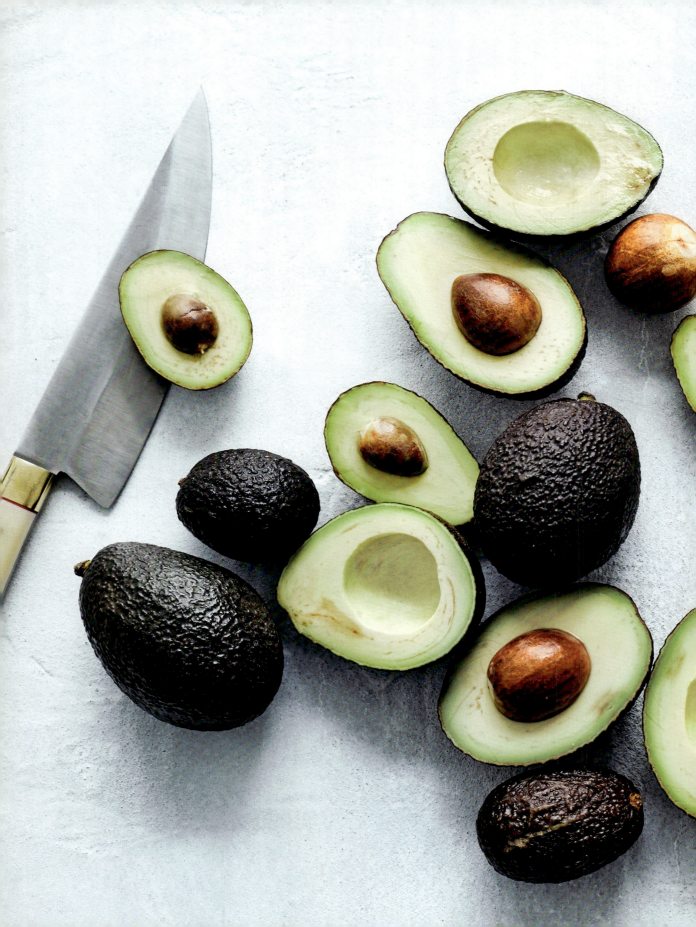

breakfast & brunch

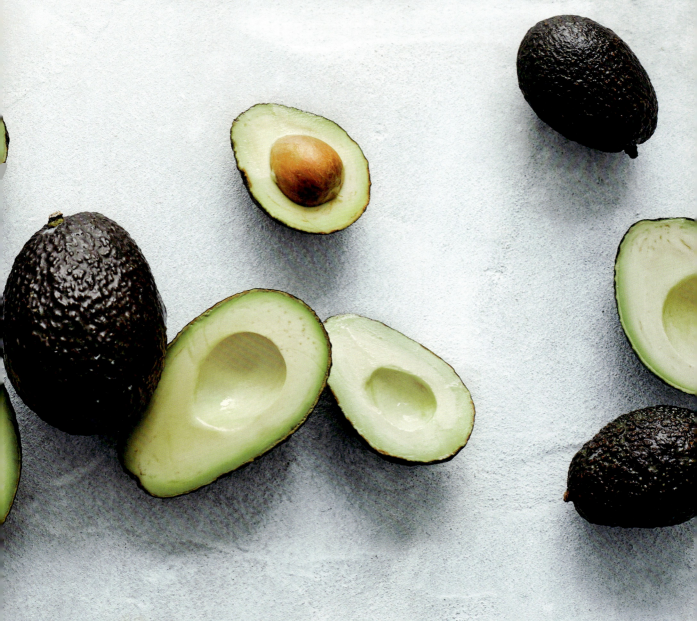

Baked Avocado Eggs

This dish, rich in monounsaturated fat and protein, provides good nutritional preparation when eaten a couple of hours before you work out. For carbs, add a slice of whole grain toast or a side of granola to your meal.

4 SERVINGS

4 slices bacon

2 avocados

1 lime, halved

Kosher salt

4 large eggs

¼ cup (15 g) minced fresh chives

Flaky sea salt, for finishing

Preheat the oven to 450°F (230°C). In a frying pan over medium heat, cook the bacon, turning as needed, until crisp, 4–6 minutes. Transfer to paper towels to drain, then crumble when cool enough to handle.

Cut each avocado in half lengthwise and remove the pit. Using a spoon, scoop out a hollow in each half just large enough to accommodate an egg (about 2 inches/5 cm in diameter). Squeeze lime juice over the flesh of each avocado half and season with kosher salt. Place the avocado halves, hollow sides up, on a baking sheet and crack an egg into each hollow.

Bake until the whites of the eggs have set but the yolks are still runny, about 12 minutes, or until done to your liking. Transfer to individual plates and garnish with the chives and bacon, dividing them evenly. Finish with a sprinkle of flaky salt, and serve.

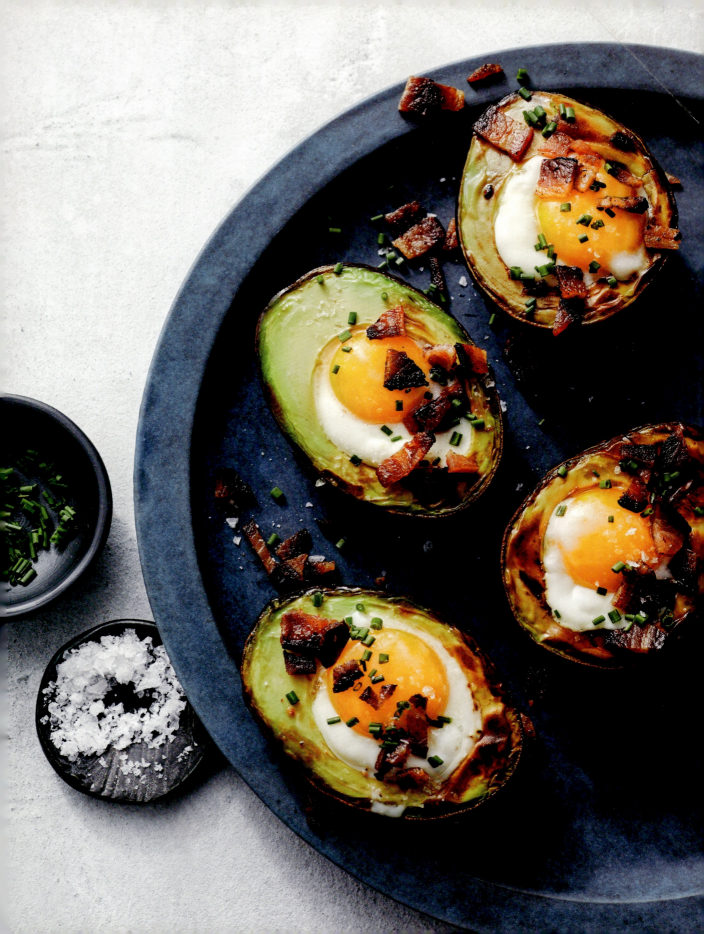

Homemade Granola with Blueberries & Yogurt

This crunchy, light granola is easy to make and lower in fat and sugar than the ones you find in stores. Wheat germ, the protein heart of whole-grain wheat, contains a wealth of micronutrients and adds a mild toasted-nut flavor. Serve it with yogurt and vitamin-packed blueberries for a strong start to the day.

6 SERVINGS

2 cups (200 g) rolled oats

½ cup (60 g) raw wheat germ

¼ cup (30 g) coarsely chopped walnuts

¼ cup (40 g) sesame seeds

¼ cup (30 g) shredded sweetened coconut

¼ cup (35 g) hulled raw pumpkin seeds

Pinch of sea salt

3 Tbsp honey

2 Tbsp avocado oil or coconut oil

1 tsp ground cinnamon

Plain Greek-style yogurt, for serving

Blueberries, for serving

  SF

Preheat the oven to 400°F (200°C). In a large bowl, combine the oats, wheat germ, walnuts, sesame seeds, coconut, pumpkin seeds, and salt and stir to mix. Spread the mixture in an even layer on a large rimmed baking sheet. Bake, stirring occasionally, until crisp and golden, about 15 minutes. Transfer to a large bowl to cool. (The cooled granola will keep at room temperature in an airtight container for up to 1 week.)

In a small saucepan over low heat, combine the honey, oil, and cinnamon and cook, stirring, just until the mixture is warm and well blended, about 2 minutes.

Add half of the honey mixture to the bowl with the granola and toss to combine and coat thoroughly. Add just enough of the remaining honey mixture so that the granola clumps slightly but is not soupy. Reserve any extra for another use.

Add a dollop of yogurt to each serving bowl. Top with a portion of granola and a small handful of blueberries, and serve right away.

Buckwheat Polenta with Blackberries

Cream of buckwheat makes a nutty-tasting hot cereal that resembles Italian polenta. It cooks in 10 minutes and doesn't need stirring. Gluten-free buckwheat has a low glycemic index that helps keep your blood sugar levels even throughout the morning. Flax adds omega-3s and minerals. Halve the recipe if cooking for one.

2 SERVINGS

1 ¼ cups (300 ml) unsweetened plain almond milk

4 Tbsp (60 ml) maple syrup

6 Tbsp (60 g) cream of buckwheat

1 ½ Tbsp ground flaxseed

1 tsp ground cinnamon

½ tsp sea salt

4 Tbsp (25 g) toasted sliced almonds (see Tip)

1 cup (145 g) fresh blackberries

In a small saucepan over medium-high heat, combine the almond milk, 2 Tbsp of the maple syrup, and 1 ¼ cups (300 ml) water and bring just to a boil. Mix in the buckwheat, flaxseed, cinnamon, and salt. Reduce the heat and simmer, stirring occasionally, until the cereal resembles creamy polenta, about 10 minutes.

Meanwhile, in a small bowl, combine the blackberries and remaining 2 Tbsp maple syrup, and with a fork mash the berries lightly. Divide the cereal between two cereal bowls and sprinkle with the almonds. Spoon the berries and syrup over the cereal. Serve right away.

TIP *To preserve freshness, toast nuts and seeds just before you are ready to use them. Preheat the oven to 350°F (180°C). Spread the nuts or seeds in a single layer on a small rimmed baking sheet and toast, stirring occasionally, until fragrant, 2–10 minutes for seeds and 5–15 minutes for nuts. The timing will vary depending on the type or size; check regularly to avoid burning.*

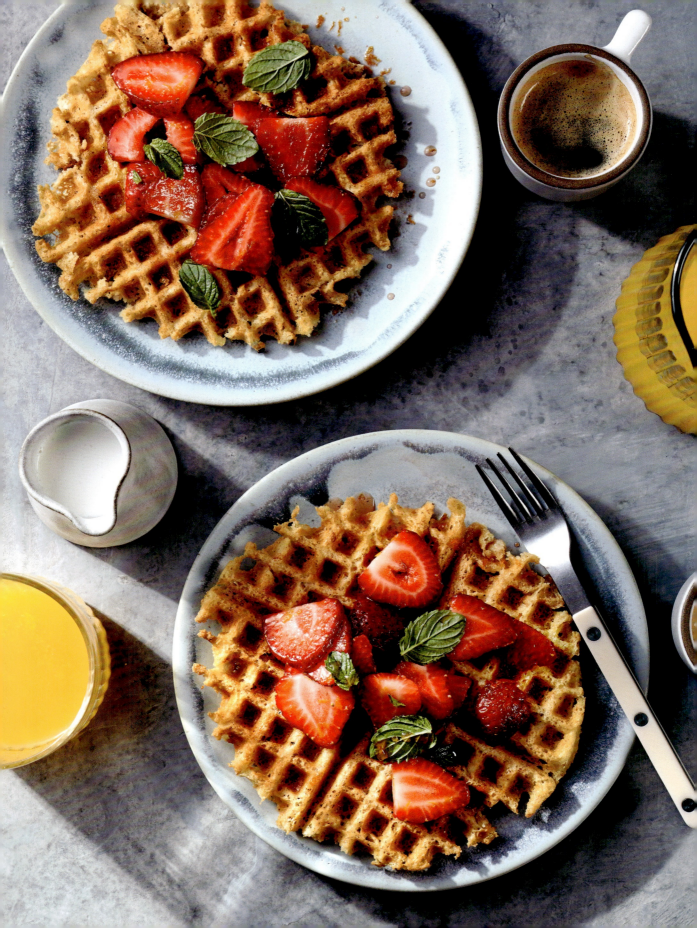

Whole-Wheat Waffles with Honeyed Strawberries

Cinnamon-flavored whole-wheat batter produces waffles with a crunchy texture and a nutty taste. They're irresistible topped with antioxidant-packed, honey-sweetened berries. Commercial growers use toxic chemicals to protect conventionally grown strawberries so consider buying organic fresh or frozen berries. Try these waffles topped with Warm Berry Compote (page 187).

4 SERVINGS

FOR THE HONEYED
STRAWBERRIES

¼ cup (60 ml) orange blossom
or wildflower honey

2 Tbsp fresh lemon juice

1 cup (125 g) hulled and sliced
strawberries

1 cup (115 g) whole-wheat flour

½ cup (60 g) unbleached
all-purpose flour

2 Tbsp wheat bran

1 Tbsp baking powder

1 tsp ground cinnamon

½ tsp fine sea salt

1 ½ cups (350 ml) milk

2 large eggs

2 Tbsp avocado oil or coconut oil

2 Tbsp wildflower or orange
blossom honey

Fresh mint leaves, for garnish
(optional)

To make the honeyed strawberries, in a small saucepan over low heat, heat the honey, stirring, until thinned but not hot, about 1 minute. Remove from the heat. Add the lemon juice and strawberries and stir until blended. Cover and let stand at room temperature until ready to serve.

In a large bowl, whisk together the flours, bran, baking powder, cinnamon, and salt. In a large glass measuring pitcher, whisk together the milk, eggs, and oil until blended. Add the 2 Tbsp honey to the milk mixture and whisk until blended. Make a well in the center of the dry ingredients and add the milk mixture. Stir just until blended; do not overmix. The batter will be thick.

Preheat the oven to 200°F (90°C) and set a heatproof platter in the oven. Preheat a nonstick waffle iron according to the manufacturer's instructions. Ladle about ½ cup (125 ml) of batter in a spiral from the outside edges in. Close the waffle iron and cook until the steam stops escaping from the sides and the top opens easily, 4–5 minutes, or according to the manufacturer's instructions. Transfer the waffle to the platter in the oven to keep warm. Repeat with the remaining batter.

Serve the waffles with the honeyed strawberries. Garnish each serving with fresh mint leaves, if desired.

Double Almond Gluten-Free Waffles with Fresh Berry Salsa

Almond flour and flax meal make these waffles higher in protein, significantly lower in carbs, and richer in fiber than those made with wheat flour. They are more tender if you use the fine almond flour made from blanched almonds rather than the brown-flecked meal made from whole almonds. Nut oils rich in the best kind of fat add flavor. Serve leftovers topped with fruit spread or almond butter for a sustaining snack.

4 SERVINGS

FOR THE FRESH BERRY SALSA

2 cups (250 g) fresh berries such as hulled and sliced strawberries, blueberries, raspberries, blackberries, or a mix

¼ cup (60 ml) maple syrup

1 cup (115 g) fine blanched almond flour

2 Tbsp ground flax seed

1 Tbsp sugar

2 tsp baking powder

Pinch of salt

⅔ cup (160 ml) unsweetened plain almond milk

1 large egg

1 Tbsp almond or avocado oil

1 Tbsp walnut or avocado oil

1 tsp pure vanilla extract

To make the berry salsa, in a mixing bowl, combine the berries and maple syrup. Mix gently and set aside for 10 minutes to let the berries give up some juice. Let stand at room temperature until ready to serve. (Use the salsa within 2 hours.)

In a large bowl, combine the almond flour, flax seed, sugar, baking powder, and salt.

In a large glass measuring pitcher, whisk together the almond milk, egg, and both oils. Pour the almond milk mixture into the dry ingredients. Whisk just until blended; do not overmix. Set the batter aside for 10 minutes; the batter will thicken to the texture of buttermilk.

Preheat the oven to 200°F (90°C) and set a heatproof platter in the oven. Preheat a nonstick mini or full size waffle iron according to the manufacturer's instructions. Ladle about ½ cup (125 ml) of batter in a spiral from the outside edges in. Close the waffle iron and cook until the top opens easily, 8–10 minutes, or according to the manufacturer's instructions. Transfer the waffle to the platter in the oven to keep warm. Repeat with the remaining batter.

Serve the waffles accompanied by the berry salsa.

Farmers' Market Scramble

Scrambling eggs with vegetables and greens is a fast and easy way to prepare a nutritious breakfast. Stir in almost any sautéed vegetables that strike your fancy, such as the tomatoes and zucchini used here. Arugula can stand in for the spinach.

4 SERVINGS

8 large eggs

2 Tbsp milk

Sea salt and freshly ground black pepper

4 tsp olive oil

1 small zucchini, trimmed and diced

1 ripe medium tomato, seeded and diced

1 cup (30 g) packed baby spinach leaves

¼ cup (1 oz/30 g) freshly grated pecorino romano cheese

In a bowl, whisk together the eggs, milk, and a pinch each of salt and pepper. Continue whisking until the eggs are nice and frothy. Set aside.

In a nonstick frying pan over medium heat, heat the olive oil. Add the zucchini and another pinch of salt. Cook, stirring, until just tender, about 1 minute. Add the tomato and stir to combine. Reduce the heat to medium-low, add the egg mixture, and let cook without stirring until the eggs just begin to set, about 1 minute. Using a heatproof rubber spatula, gently push the eggs around the pan, letting any uncooked egg run onto the bottom of the pan.

When the eggs are about half cooked, 1–2 minutes longer, add the spinach and the cheese. Fold gently to combine and continue cooking until the eggs are completely set but still moist, about 1 minute longer. Transfer the scramble to a platter and serve right away.

Peaches & Cream Breakfast Parfait

Alternating layers of cottage cheese and spiced peaches, this nutrition-packed breakfast is ready in fifteen minutes—or less, if you make its fiber-rich topping ahead. Serve it for brunch in a wineglass, or spoon the peaches into a to-go container or jar, add the cottage cheese and topping, and enjoy this breakfast on the move.

2 SERVINGS

1 tsp unsalted butter

2 Tbsp freshly squeezed orange juice

2 Tbsp honey

½ tsp ground cinnamon

¼ tsp pure vanilla extract

1 bag (10 oz/280 g) frozen unsweetened sliced peaches

1 cup (210 g) cottage cheese

1 tsp fresh lime juice

2 Tbsp Four-Seed Topping (page 187)

In a medium nonstick frying pan over medium heat, melt the butter. Off the heat, add the orange juice, honey, cinnamon, and vanilla. Return the pan to medium heat and cook, stirring, until the sauce starts to bubble, 4 minutes. Add the peaches, stir to coat them with the sauce, cover, and simmer until they are warmed through, 5 minutes. Uncover and set aside to cool slightly.

While the peaches cool, in a small bowl, combine the cottage cheese and lime juice.

When the peaches are lukewarm, spoon one-fourth of them into the bottom of each of two bowls or glasses. Add some syrup from the pan. Spoon about one-fourth of the cottage cheese mixture over the peaches in each bowl. Top with the remaining peaches and liquid from the pan. Divide the remaining cottage cheese between the bowls. At this point, the parfaits can be covered with plastic wrap and refrigerated overnight, if desired. Before serving, sprinkle half of the four seed topping over each bowl and serve right away.

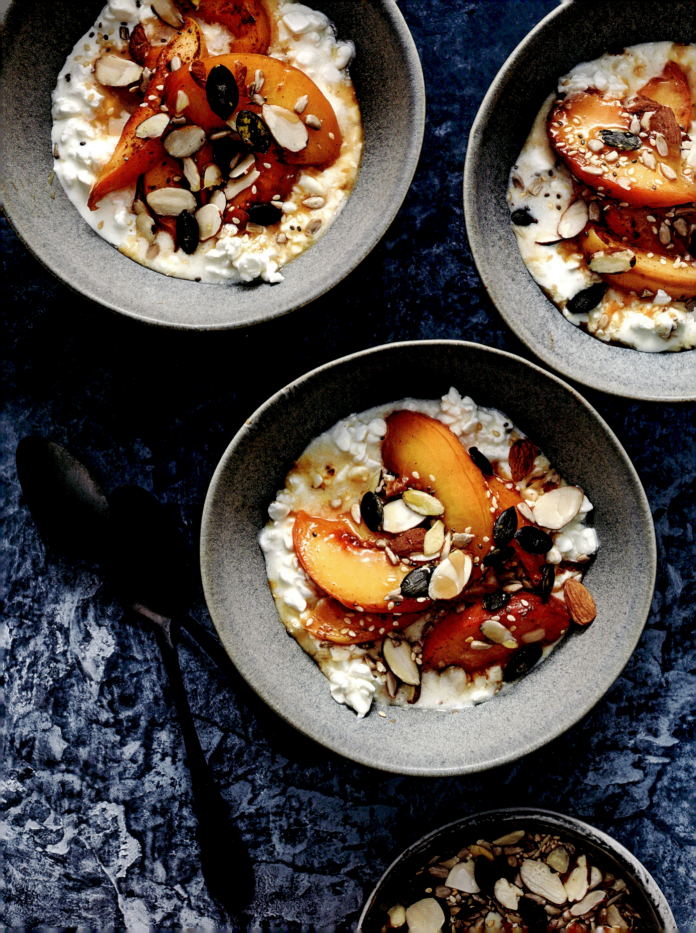

Loaded Avocado Toast

This avocado toast makes a satisfying yet light meal combining healthy fats and protein with the bright acidity of tomatoes and the peppery bite of crunchy radishes. Served for breakfast, this is a good way to start your day on the right foot.

1 SERVING

1 clove garlic, lightly smashed

1 thick slice coarse country bread, toasted

½ avocado, halved, pitted, and sliced

Flaky sea salt and freshly ground black pepper

1 hard-cooked egg, peeled and thinly sliced (see Tip)

1 radish, thinly sliced

¼ cup (60 g) multicolor cherry tomatoes, halved

Rub the garlic clove over one side of the toasted bread slice. Arrange the avocado slices in an even layer on the garlic-rubbed bread, then use a fork to smash the avocado evenly over the entire surface. Season with salt. Arrange the egg slices, radish slices, and tomatoes on top, in an appealing pattern. Sprinkle with more salt, finish with pepper, and serve.

TIP *To hard cook eggs, place in a saucepan with enough water to cover by 1 inch (2.5 cm). Bring to a boil over medium-high heat. Remove the pan from the heat, cover, and let stand until done to your liking, about 10 minutes for slightly runny yolks and up to 14 minutes for firm yolks. Drain the eggs, then transfer to a bowl of ice water to cool slightly, 2 minutes or so.*

Carrot Breakfast Muffins

These whole-grain muffins are surprisingly moist and light. Combining carrots, raisins, walnuts, and whole-wheat flour, they are fiber-rich in the nicest way. The topping of seeds and nuts brings appealing crunch. Enjoy one for breakfast and tuck a second muffin away as an afternoon snack.

12 MUFFINS

1 cup (115 g) whole-wheat flour

1 cup (115 g) unbleached all-purpose flour

1 Tbsp baking powder

½ tsp baking soda

½ cup (100 g) firmly packed brown sugar

1 tsp ground cinnamon

¼ tsp sea salt

1 cup (150 g) raisins

1 cup (120 g) chopped walnuts

1 ½ cups (180 g) shredded carrot

1 cup (240 ml) buttermilk

⅓ cup (75 ml) avocado oil or coconut oil

1 large egg

Spicy Seed Sprinkle (page 159)

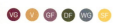

Preheat the oven to 400°F (200°C). Coat the 12 cups of a standard muffin pan with cooking spray, or use paper liners.

In a large bowl, whisk together the two flours, baking powder, baking soda, brown sugar, cinnamon, and salt. Add the raisins, walnuts, and carrots and toss with your hands to coat with the dry ingredients and distribute them evenly.

In a large measuring cup, whisk together the buttermilk, oil, and egg until they are blended. Pour the wet ingredients into the dry ingredients and stir just until blended. Do not overmix. Spoon the batter into the prepared muffin cups, dividing it evenly. Top each muffin with an equal amount of the seed sprinkle.

Bake the muffins until they are lightly browned and a toothpick inserted into the center comes out clean, 20–25 minutes. Let cool in the pan on a wire rack for 5 minutes, then turn out the muffins onto the rack and let cool for 10 minutes longer. Serve warm. Or, let the muffins cool completely and store in a resealable plastic bag at room temperature for up to 3 days.

Poached Eggs with White Bean & Tomato Ragout

White beans simmered with fire-roasted tomatoes and rosemary make an enticing base for poached eggs and add micronutrients to round out the eggs' protein and fats. It's a novel and satisfying choice for a morning meal. The beans alone make a delicious side dish served to accompany chicken, lamb, or pork. A sprinkling of grated cheese would be a nice addition, try Manchego or a sheep's milk pecorino helpful for the lactose-sensitive. Serve with thick slices of grilled country bread.

4 SERVINGS

1 Tbsp olive oil

2 thick slices pancetta (about 3 oz/90 g total weight), chopped (optional)

1 large yellow onion, finely chopped

4 tsp minced fresh rosemary

¼–½ tsp red chile flakes

2 cans (14.5 oz/411 g each) fire-roasted tomatoes

2 cans (15 oz/425 g each) cannellini beans, drained and rinsed

Kosher salt and freshly ground black pepper

1–2 tsp white wine vinegar

4–8 large eggs

Freshly grated Parmesan cheese, for serving

In a large saucepan over medium heat, heat the oil. Add the chopped pancetta, if using, and sauté until it starts to brown, about 3 minutes. Add the onion, rosemary, and red chile flakes, and sauté until the onion is tender, about 5 minutes.

Add the tomatoes with their juices and the beans. Mix in ¾ cup (180 ml) water. Bring to a boil, reduce the heat, and simmer until the mixture thickens and the flavors blend, about 15 minutes. Season to taste with salt and pepper.

Meanwhile, pour water into 1 (for 4 eggs) or 2 (for 8 eggs) large frying pans to the depth of 1 inch (2.5 cm). Season the water with salt and add 1 tsp vinegar to each frying pan. Bring the liquid to a boil, and then reduce the heat to maintain a bare simmer. One at a time, break an egg into a small cup, and then gently slip into the water. Simmer gently until the eggs are cooked as desired, 3–4 minutes for runny yolks or up to 5 minutes for firmer yolks.

Divide the white bean mixture among serving bowls. Using a slotted spoon, transfer 1 or 2 eggs to each bowl. Top the eggs with grated cheese, if using, and black pepper and serve right away.

TIP *Fire-roasted canned tomatoes are a flavorful convenience item to keep on hand in the pantry.*

Brussels Sprouts with Potato Hash & Baked Eggs

Serving breakfast for dinner always wins praise, and you can feel good about this dish because it's loaded with vegetables along with high-protein eggs. Keep in mind that the eggs will continue to cook from the residual heat after you remove the pan from the oven.

4 SERVINGS

1 ¼ lb (625 g) Brussels sprouts

2 russet potatoes, unpeeled, cut into ¼-inch (6-mm) pieces

3 tablespoons fresh thyme leaves, roughly chopped

2 shallots, halved and sliced

2 cloves garlic, chopped

½ cup (125 ml) olive oil, plus more as needed

Kosher salt and freshly ground black pepper

8 large eggs

Hot sauce, for serving (optional)

Preheat the oven to 425°F (220°C). Line a sheet pan with aluminum foil.

Trim the ends off the Brussels sprouts, halve them lengthwise, and then coarsely chop into small dice. They will fall apart, and this is fine.

Transfer the Brussels sprouts to a large bowl. Add the potatoes, thyme, shallots, garlic, and oil and stir to combine.

Place the vegetables in a single layer on the prepared pan and season generously with salt and pepper. Roast for 15 minutes, then stir the vegetables and spread them out in a single layer again. Drizzle with more oil if they seem dry. Continue roasting until the vegetables are golden and fork tender, about 15 minutes longer.

Using a spoon, make 8 small wells for the eggs in the vegetables. Crack 1 egg into each well and season with salt and pepper. Bake until the eggs are mostly set, 6–8 minutes.

To serve, carefully scoop 2 eggs and some of the hash into each of 4 bowls. Serve right away with hot sauce, if using.

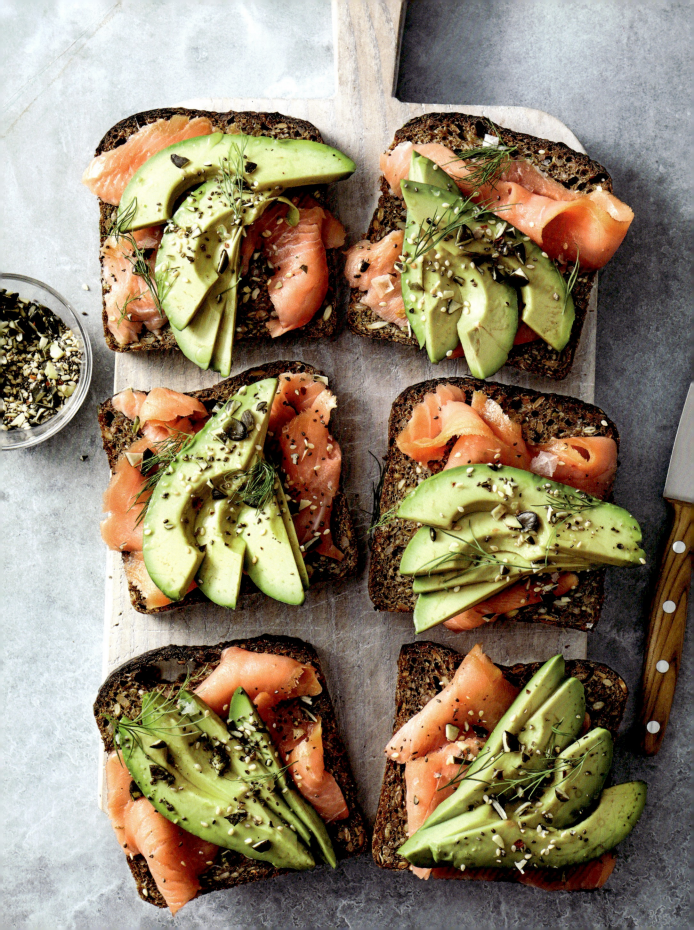

Smoked Salmon & Avocado Tartine with Spicy Seed Sprinkle

Smoked salmon, avocado, and a blend of nuts and seeds topping thin slices of traditional Scandinavian or German dark rye bread make a light meal that is rich in beneficial fiber, hunger-banishing protein, and healthy fat. The spicy seed topping also adds spark to salads or an almond butter sandwich. It is also surprisingly good on your morning oatmeal!

4 SERVINGS

8 square slices Scandinavian-style dark rye bread

16 slices smoked salmon (about 16 oz/500 g)

2 ripe small avocados, halved, pitted, and quartered

2 tsp fresh lime juice

Sea salt

2 Tbsp extra-virgin olive oil

FOR THE SPICY SEED SPRINKLE

8 toasted almonds, chopped

2 tsp raw pumpkin seeds, coarsely chopped

1 tsp chia seeds

1 tsp toasted sesame seeds, white or black

Pinch of red chile flakes

Sea salt (optional)

DF WG SF

On each of the 8 squares of bread, arrange 2 salmon slices. For each tartine, scoop an avocado quarter from the peel, cut it into 4 long slices, and arrange the slices on top of the salmon.

In a small bowl, whisk together the lime juice, a pinch of salt, and the olive oil. Drizzle 1 tsp of the lime mixture over each tartine.

To make the spicy seed sprinkle, in another small bowl, combine the almonds, pumpkin seeds, chia seeds, sesame seeds, and red chile flakes. Season with salt, if desired. Top each tartine with 1 tsp of the spicy seed sprinkle. Serve right away.

Asparagus, Goat Cheese & Chive Omelet

When you need a morning meal that will keep you full and focused for hours, this omelet does the trick. Here, grassy, vitamin-rich asparagus brightens under a tangy crumble of goat cheese nestled in a protein-rich country-style omelet. While this dish is perfect for jump starting your day, it also makes an easy yet sophisticated supper.

2 SERVINGS

1 Tbsp olive oil

10 oz (280 g) thin asparagus, trimmed and sliced diagonally into 3-inch (7.5-cm) lengths

4 large eggs, lightly beaten

Kosher salt and freshly ground black pepper

½ cup (2 oz/60 g) crumbled fresh goat cheese

2 Tbsp minced fresh chives

In a large nonstick frying pan over medium-high heat, heat the olive oil. Add the asparagus and stir and toss constantly until lightly coated with the oil, about 1 minute. Add 2 Tbsp water, cover, and cook until the water evaporates and the asparagus is just tender, about 2 minutes.

Reduce the heat to medium and shake the pan to distribute the asparagus evenly over the bottom. Pour the eggs over the asparagus, tilting the pan to distribute them evenly but being careful not to dislodge the asparagus, and season with salt and pepper. Cook until the eggs are just set on the bottom, about 3 minutes.

Sprinkle the omelet evenly with the cheese and chives. Cover the pan and remove from the heat. Let stand until the eggs are just set and the cheese is heated through, about 3 minutes.

Loosen the omelet with a wooden spatula and slide it onto a large, flat platter. Serve warm or at room temperature.

Huevos Rancheros with Black Bean Mash & Tomatillo Salsa

Beans, high in protein and fiber but low in calories, make an excellent breakfast option for those focusing on weight loss. If watching your sodium intake, be sure to select low-sodium beans, as they cut the dish's sodium content by more than half. You can use one (15.4-oz) can of refried beans as a time-saving substitute for the black bean mash.

4 SERVINGS

1 ½ lb (680 g) tomatillos, husked, rinsed, and halved

1 white onion, quartered

3 cloves garlic, unpeeled

1 serrano chile, halved lengthwise

5 Tbsp (75 ml) avocado oil or coconut oil

½ cup (20 g) packed fresh cilantro leaves, plus more for serving

1 Tbsp fresh lime juice

Kosher salt

8 taco-sized corn tortillas

4 large eggs

Black Bean Mash (page 185)

Queso fresco and flaky sea salt, for serving

Position a rack in the upper third of the oven and preheat the broiler. Pile the tomatillos, onion quarters, garlic cloves, and serrano on a baking sheet, drizzle with 2 Tbsp of the oil, and toss to coat. Spread the vegetables on the pan, arranging the tomatillos, onion, and chile cut-side down, and broil until charred and softened, about 10 minutes. Remove from the oven and let the garlic cloves cool until they can be handled, then peel them.

Transfer the tomatillos, onion, serrano, and garlic to a food processor, add the cilantro, and pulse until a salsa-like texture is achieved. Stir in the lime juice and season to taste with kosher salt.

Have ready a sheet of aluminum foil. In a nonstick frying pan over high heat, heat 1 Tbsp of the oil. Add the tortillas, one at a time, and fry, turning once, until the edges begin to crisp, about 30 seconds per side, then transfer to the foil. Wrap the tortillas in the foil to keep warm until serving.

In the same pan, reduce the heat to medium-high and add the remaining 2 Tbsp oil. Crack the eggs into the pan and cook until the whites are set but the yolks remain runny, about 4 minutes, or until done to your liking.

To serve, place 2 toasted tortillas on each individual plate and spread with the refried beans. Top each serving with an egg, spoon the tomatillo salsa all around, and garnish with the queso fresco, cilantro leaves, and flaky sea salt.

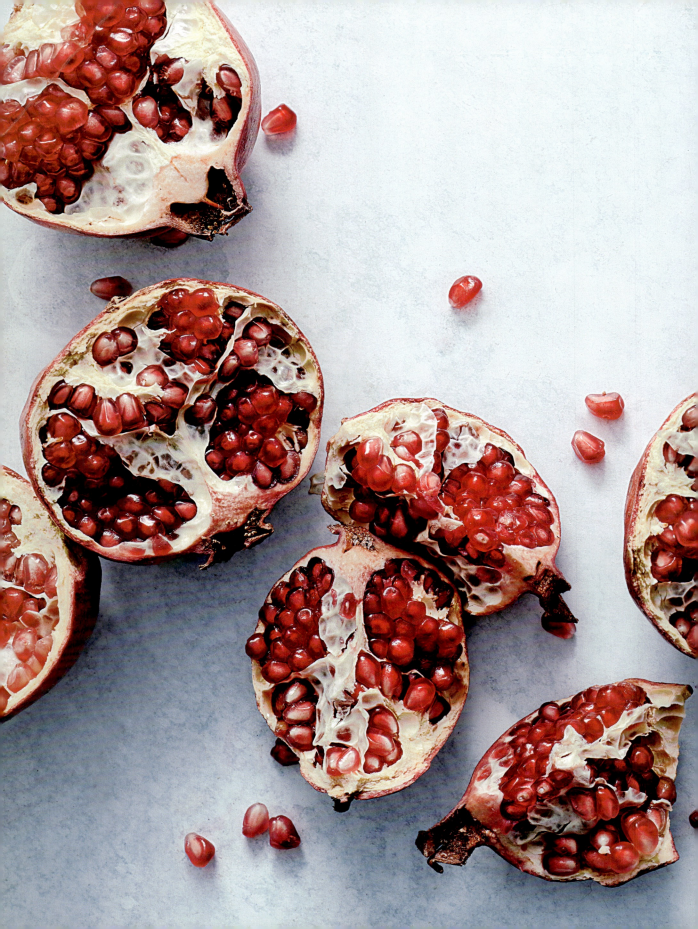

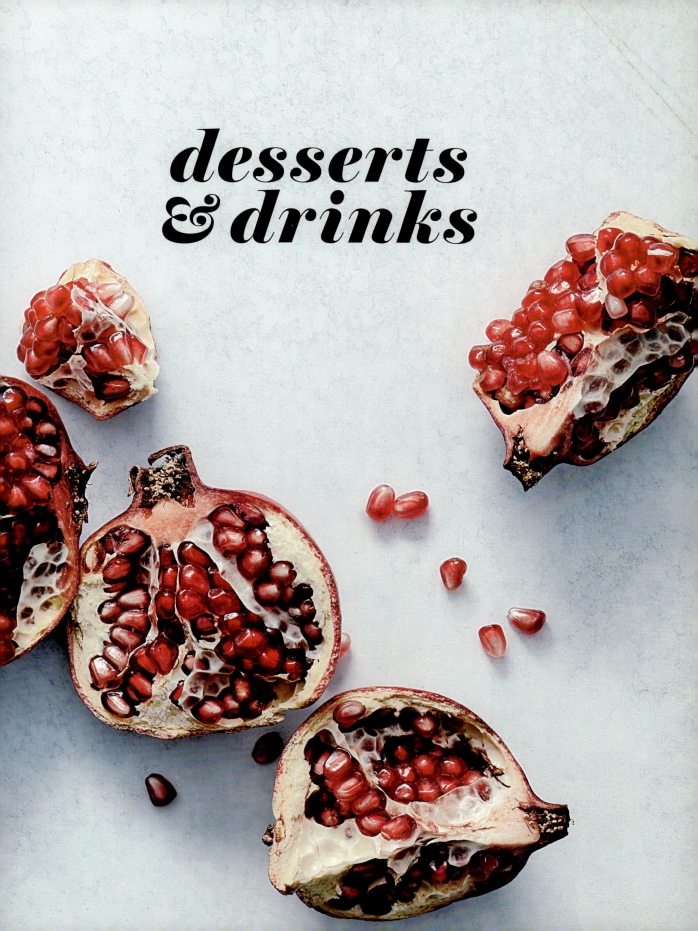

desserts
& drinks

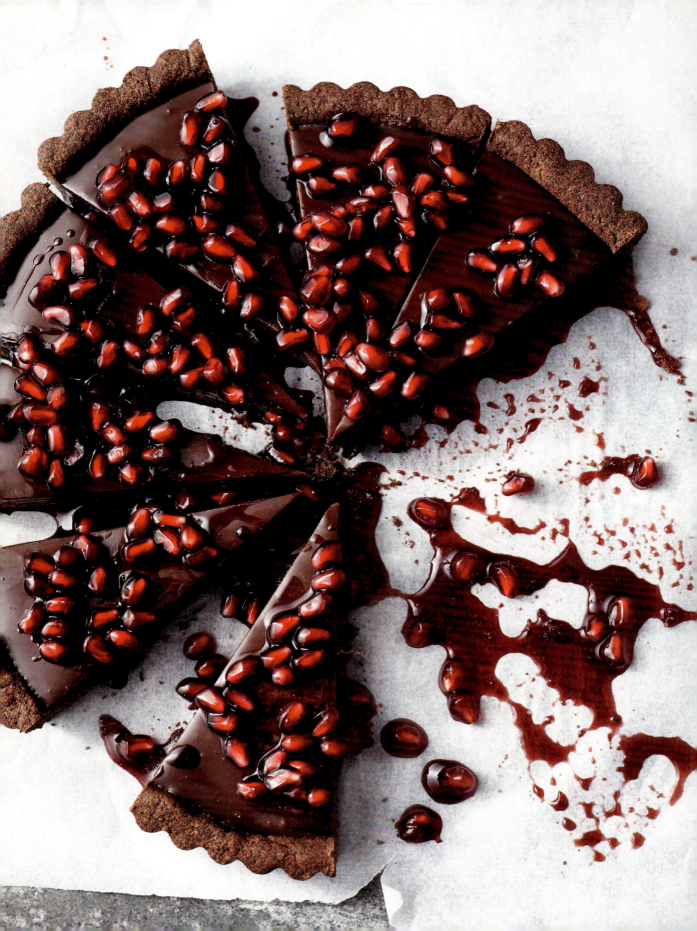

Chocolate Tart with Buckwheat Crust & Pomegranate Glaze

This elegant tart is a delicious as it is nutritious, with high micronutrient content and loads of fiber. Despite the name, buckwheat is not related to wheat and is free of gluten.

10–12 SERVINGS

FOR THE CRUST

1 ⅓ cups (160 g) buckwheat flour

¼ cup (30 g) cornstarch

½ cup (40 g) Dutch process cocoa powder

⅓ cup plus 2 Tbsp (30 g) sugar

½ tsp sea salt

½ cup (115 g) cold unsalted butter, cut into cubes

1 tsp pure vanilla extract

4–6 Tbsp (60–90 ml) cold water

FOR THE FILLING

12 oz (340 g) dark chocolate, chopped

1 ¼ cups (300 ml) heavy cream

½ tsp pure vanilla extract

FOR THE GLAZE

2 cups (475 ml) pomegranate juice

¼ cup (50 g) sugar

2 pomegranates, seeded (about 1 cup/140 g seeds)

FOR THE WHIP

1 cup (250 ml) heavy cream

¼ cup (60 g) mascarpone cheese, at room temperature

To make the crust, preheat the oven to 350°F (180°C). In a food processor, combine the flour, cornstarch, cocoa powder, sugar, and salt and process just until combined, about 10 seconds. Scatter the butter over the flour mixture and pulse until the mixture has the texture of sand. Add the vanilla and 4 tablespoons (60 ml) of the water and pulse just until the dough comes together in a rough mass. Pinch a little of the dough between your fingers; if it doesn't hold together, gradually pulse in 1–2 tablespoons more water.

Transfer the dough to a 9-inch (23-cm) tart pan with a removable bottom and press it evenly onto the bottom and up the sides of the pan. Prick the bottom all over with a fork, then refrigerate the crust for 30 minutes.

Bake the crust until slightly puffed and darkened, 15–17 minutes. Remove from the oven and let cool completely on a wire rack.

To make the filling, put the chocolate in a heatproof bowl. In a small saucepan over medium heat, bring the cream just to a boil. Immediately pour the cream over the chocolate and let stand for 2 minutes. Add the vanilla and whisk until the mixture is well blended and smooth. Pour the filling into the cooled crust, cover, and chill for at least 3 hours or up to overnight.

To make the glaze, in a small saucepan over high heat, combine the pomegranate juice and sugar and bring to a boil, stirring to dissolve the sugar. Reduce the heat to low and cook, stirring, until the mixture has reduced by half and coats the back of a spoon, about 20 minutes. Remove from the heat, fold in the pomegranate seeds, and let cool completely. Pour the glaze evenly over the surface of the chilled tart.

To make the whip, in a bowl, using a handheld mixer, beat the cream on medium-high speed until soft peaks form when the whisk is lifted. Add the mascarpone and continue to beat until combined and the soft peaks hold.

Remove the pan sides and place the tart on a serving plate. Cut into wedges and garnish each serving with the whip.

Chocolate Avocado Mousse with Coconut Cream

The creamy avocado and the chocolate in this divine dessert are rich in micronutrient and healthy fat. Chocolate is high in iron and antioxidants. Dark chocolate in particular can help ease hypertension thanks to its flavanols, helpful organic chemicals found in plants. The darker the chocolate, the more flavanols and less sugar it may contain.

4–6 SERVINGS

FOR THE AVOCADO MOUSSE

5 oz (150 g) dark chocolate, coarsely chopped

2 avocados, halved and pitted

¾ cup (65 g) Dutch-process cocoa powder

⅓ cup (75 ml) unsweetened almond milk

⅓ cup (70 g) plus 2 Tbsp granulated sugar

2 tsp pure vanilla extract

½ tsp sea salt

FOR THE COCONUT CREAM

1 can (14 fl oz/400 ml) coconut milk, well chilled and unshaken

½ cup (50 g) confectioners' sugar

½ tsp pure vanilla extract

2 oz (60 g) dark chocolate, coarsely chopped, for garnish

½ cup (60 g) cocoa nibs, for garnish

Blackberries and sliced strawberries, for garnish (optional)

To make the avocado mousse, put the chocolate in a microwaveable bowl and heat in 30-second increments until the chocolate is almost but not completely melted. Stir with a heat-resistant spatula until completely melted and smooth. Let cool.

In a food processor, combine the scooped-out avocado flesh, melted chocolate (set the bowl aside unwashed), the cocoa powder, almond milk, granulated sugar, vanilla, and salt and process until very smooth, about 2 minutes, stopping and scraping down the sides of the bowl as needed. Transfer to a small bowl and refrigerate for 30 minutes.

Meanwhile, make the coconut cream. Open the can of coconut milk and scoop off the firm, thick layer of cream solidified on top, dropping it into the bowl of a stand mixer fitted with the whisk attachment. Reserve the remainder of the contents for another use. Add the confectioners' sugar and vanilla to the mixer and whip on high speed until medium-firm peaks form when the whisk is lifted, about 3 minutes. Cover and refrigerate for 30 minutes.

Using the unwashed bowl, melt the chocolate for garnish the same way as before, and let cool to room temperature.

To serve, spoon the avocado mousse into individual bowls and top with the coconut cream, a drizzle of melted chocolate, and a sprinkling of cocoa nibs. Top with a few berries, if using.

Dark Chocolate Banana Bites with Roasted Almonds

Naturally sweet and creamy when frozen, bananas are rich in potassium. Coated with dark chocolate and nuts they make a super healthy treat. Choose bright yellow bananas with just a bit of speckling—they will have some firmness and be easier to handle than fully ripe ones.

ABOUT 30 BITES;
6–8 SERVINGS

12 oz (350 g) bittersweet chocolate, chopped

⅔ cup (90 g) roasted almonds or pecans, chopped

2 ripe bananas

In a bowl set over a pan of barely simmering water, melt the chocolate, stirring occasionally, until smooth. Remove the pan from the heat, but leave the bowl of chocolate on top to keep warm. Put the nuts in a small bowl. Line a baking sheet with waxed paper.

Peel the bananas and cut them into ½-inch (12-mm) rounds. Drop 1 banana slice at a time into the chocolate and turn to coat. Lift out with a fork, tapping the fork gently on the bowl edge to allow excess chocolate to drip back into the bowl. Place the banana slice on the prepared baking sheet and sprinkle with nuts. Repeat to dip and coat the remaining banana slices.

Freeze the coated bananas until the chocolate is set, about 20 minutes, then transfer to an airtight container and store in the freezer for up to 1 week.

Coconut Macaroons

If you want to eat less gluten, flourless coconut macaroons are the cookie for you. For a variation, dip the bottoms of the macaroons in melted dark chocolate, return them to the parchment-lined pan, and refrigerate until the chocolate is set.

48 COOKIES

3 large egg whites,
at room temperature

¼ tsp cream of tartar

Kosher salt

¾ cup (150 g) sugar

½ tsp pure vanilla extract

4 ½ cups (10 oz/150 g)
sweetened shredded coconut

Preheat the oven to 325°F (160°C). Line 3 baking sheets with parchment paper. In a large bowl, combine the egg whites and cream of tartar. Using a mixer on medium-high speed, beat until the egg whites are very foamy, about 1 minute. Add a pinch of salt. While beating continuously, gradually add the sugar and beat until stiff peaks form when the whisk is lifted, 3–4 minutes.

Using a rubber spatula, stir in the vanilla. In 3 batches, gently fold the coconut into the beaten whites just until incorporated. Place rounded tablespoonfuls of the dough 1 ½ inches (4 cm) apart on the prepared baking sheets. Bake until the cookie edges begin to turn light golden brown, 19–22 minutes.

Let the cookies cool completely on the sheets, about 30 minutes. Store in a single layer in an airtight container at room temperature for up to 4 days.

Pistachio Olive Oil Torte

This rustic cake manages to be moist, chewy, and, thanks to the polenta, delicately crunchy all at once. It's not too sweet, making it a good breakfast choice as well as dessert. It also happens to be gluten free!

8–10 SERVINGS

Olive oil spray

1 ½ cups (150 g) plus ¼ cup (25 g) shelled unsalted pistachios

1 cup (185 g) stone-ground cornmeal or polenta

1 tsp baking powder

½ tsp kosher salt

¾ cup (150 grams) superfine sugar

3 large eggs

¾ cup (180 ml) olive oil

Whipped cream, rice whip, yogurt, or crème fraîche, for serving

2 cups (250 g) strawberries, hulled and sliced, for serving

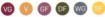

Preheat the oven to 350°F (180°C) and set a rack in the center of the oven. Line a 9-inch (23-cm) round cake pan with parchment paper and spray with olive oil spray.

Put the 1 ½ cups (150 g) pistachios in a food processor and pulse until ground to the consistency of almond meal. Roughly chop the ¼ cup (25 g) pistachios and set aside.

Sift together the cornmeal, baking powder, and salt.

Using a stand mixer fitted with the whisk attachment, beat the sugar and eggs together on medium-high speed until pale and fluffy, about 5 minutes. With the mixer running, add the olive oil, mixing until thoroughly combined.

Using a rubber spatula, gently fold in the ground pistachios and the cornmeal mixture. Scrape the batter into the prepared cake pan. Scatter the chopped pistachios over the top.

Bake until the torte is golden, the sides of the cake are just starting to pull away from the walls of the pan, and a cake tester inserted in the center comes out clean, 45–50 minutes.

Transfer the torte to a cooling rack and let cool to room temperature. Place a plate over the cake pan, invert both and shake gently to release the cake from the pan, then use a second plate to carefully flip it back over so the nut-strewn side is facing up again. Serve with whipped cream and sliced strawberries.

Grilled Peaches with Honey & Black Pepper

Peaches and nectarines are both at their peak from early through midsummer. Both come in freestone and clingstone varieties, referring to how loosely or tightly the fruit's silken flesh holds onto its large pit. Freestones are much easier for cutting and cooking; clingstones are good for eating out of hand. Both can have yellow or white flesh. Yellow indicates the presence of valuable antioxidants that are also pigments. The higher acid in yellow varieties also makes them richer in vitamin C. White varieties are sweeter, softer, and more aromatic.

4 SERVINGS

Avocado or olive oil

¼ cup (85 g) honey

Sea salt and freshly ground black pepper

4 firm but ripe peaches or nectarines, halved and pitted

Greek yogurt, rice whip, or vanilla ice cream, for serving

Prepare a grill for direct-heat cooking over medium-high heat, or use a stove-top grill pan. Oil the grill grate or pan.

In a small bowl, combine the honey, a pinch of salt, and 1 tsp pepper. Brush the peach halves with oil and place on the grill rack, cut-side down. Cover and cook until the peaches just begin to soften, 3–4 minutes. Turn the peaches and brush with the honey mixture. Cook until tender but not falling apart, 2–3 minutes longer.

Serve right away, accompanied by a dollop of yogurt.

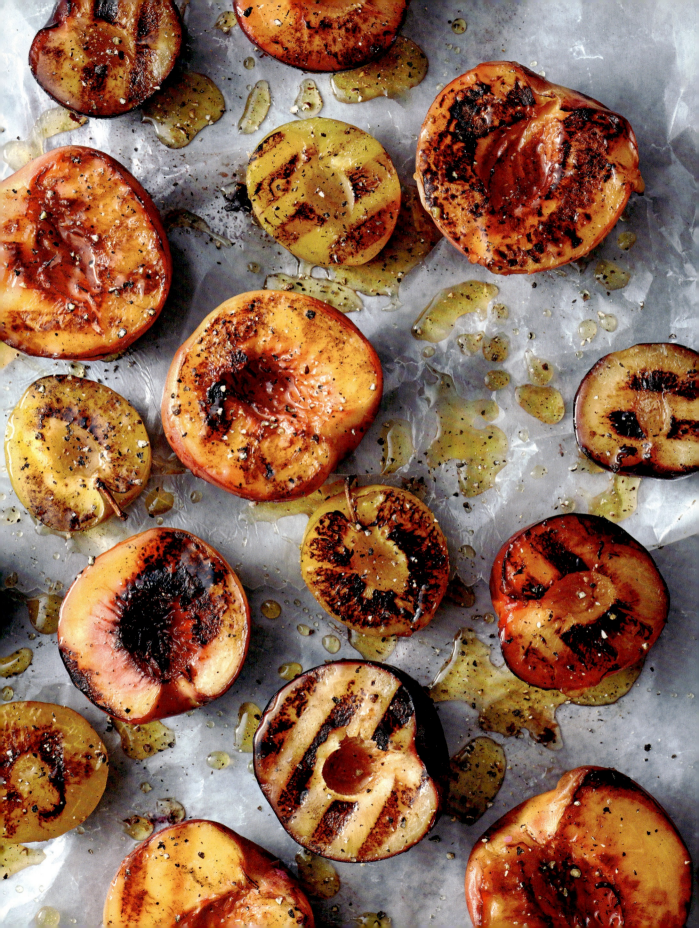

Apple-Cranberry Crumble

In fall, as the weather cools, we crave no-fuss desserts made with the season's bounty. Here, tart green apples—heirloom Newtown Pippin and Rhode Island Greening as well as familiar Granny Smith—are good choices to bake to tenderness under an oat-flecked golden topping. Dried cranberries add color and flavor along with useful micronutrients.

6–8 SERVINGS

1 ¼ cups (145 g) unbleached all-purpose flour

¾ cup (75 g) rolled oats

¾ cup (160 g) firmly packed light brown sugar

1 ½ tsp grated lemon zest

2 tsp ground cinnamon

½ tsp freshly grated nutmeg

¼ tsp sea salt

6 Tbsp (3 oz/90 g) cold unsalted butter, cut into small pieces, plus more for greasing

5 tart green apples, cored and sliced

1 Tbsp fresh lemon juice

¾ cup (90 g) dried cranberries or cherries

1 cup (200 g) granulated sugar

Vanilla ice cream, for serving (optional)

In a bowl, stir together 1 cup (115 g) of the flour, the oats, brown sugar, lemon zest, cinnamon, nutmeg, and salt. Scatter 4 Tbsp (60 g) of the butter over the top and, using your fingers, two knives, or a pastry blender, work the butter into the flour until the mixture is crumbly. Set aside.

Preheat the oven to 350°F (180°C). Lightly grease a shallow 2-qt (2-l) baking dish with butter. Place the apple slices in a large bowl, sprinkle with the lemon juice, and toss them to coat evenly. Add the cranberries, granulated sugar, and the remaining ¼ cup (30 g) flour and toss to combine. Transfer the apple mixture to the prepared baking dish and spread in an even layer. Dot the top with the remaining 2 Tbsp butter. Sprinkle the oat mixture evenly over the fruit.

Bake until the topping is browned and the juices are bubbling, about 1 hour. Serve warm or at room temperature, with the vanilla ice cream, if you like.

TIP *Trade out the apples for sliced pears—Bartlett, Anjou, Bosc, and Winter Nelis are all good bakers—and the dried cranberries for dried blueberries or dried cherries. You can also serve whipped cream, spiked with a little Calvados or brandy, if you like, in place of the ice cream.*

Dark Chocolate Pudding

This is comfort food for chocolate lovers and for everyone who loves cooking real food the old-fashioned way. It contains half the added sugar called for in classic recipes. Natural cocoa retains more of the beneficial substances that are lost when it is Dutch processed. Oat milk adds silken texture and contains about half as much healthful fiber as oatmeal, making it a good choice for a liquid.

4 SERVINGS

2 cups (475 ml) oat milk

¼ cup (50 g) firmly packed light brown sugar

2 Tbsp unsweetened natural cocoa power

2 Tbsp cornstarch

¼ tsp ground cinnamon

Pinch of sea salt

2 oz (60 g) bittersweet (70–73 percent cacao) chocolate, finely chopped

1 tsp pure vanilla extract

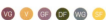

In a heatproof measuring cup in the microwave, or a small saucepan over medium heat, heat 1 ¾ cups (425 ml) of the milk until bubbles form in a ring around the edge. Set the hot milk aside.

In a heavy medium saucepan, whisk together the brown sugar, cocoa powder, cornstarch, cinnamon, and salt. Whisk in the remaining ¼ cup (50 ml) cold milk. While whisking, slowly add the hot milk to the chocolate mixture. Set the pot over medium heat and cook, whisking often, until the pudding is thick enough for your finger to leave a line on the back of a wooden spoon dipped into it, about 5 minutes. Do not let the pudding boil.

Off the heat, add the chopped chocolate and whisk until it is melted. Stir in the vanilla. Return the pudding to the heat and cook, stirring, until it is very thick, about 1 minute. Divide the hot pudding among 4 pudding cups or small bowls. To avoid a skin forming, press plastic wrap onto the surface of each serving. Let cool, then serve the pudding lukewarm or at room temperature, or refrigerate until chilled, about 3 hours, before serving. The pudding will keep for 4 days, covered, in the refrigerator.

TIP *Look for oat milk in shelf-stable packages at well-stocked supermarkets, or order it online.*

Lemony Avocado Sorbet

When you have a couple of really ripe avocados, whirl up this chilled dessert. Lemon juice brings refreshing tartness, while the zest adds unexpected depth of flavor. The great aroma and bright color in all citrus zest come from compounds that also happen to be super good for you, nutritionally speaking. For a vegan option, use nondairy milk to make this elegant sorbet.

4 SERVINGS

2 cups (230 g) halved, pitted, and diced ripe avocado (about 2 small avocados)

½ cup (50 g) confectioners' sugar

1 cup (250 ml) whole milk or oat milk

1 lemon, zested with a grater and juiced

In a food processor, combine the avocado, sugar, milk, lemon zest to taste, and the lemon juice, and whirl until puréed. Transfer the avocado mixture to a medium bowl and cover with plastic wrap, pressing the wrap onto the surface of the purée, and refrigerate until very cold, 4–8 hours.

Pour the chilled mixture into an ice-cream maker and freeze according to the manufacturer's instructions. Spoon the sorbet into a freezer-safe container and place parchment paper or waxed paper directly on top. Cover tightly and freeze until firm, at least 2 hours and up to 24 hours. The sorbet is best served within 24 hours.

Tahini-Chocolate Ice Pops

A chocoholic's delight, these frozen fudge bars are loaded with the antioxidants found in cacao. Tahini makes them creamy and brings a touch of toasty flavor. It adds calcium, as well. Pouring hot milk over the chocolate to melt it removes the risk of its burning or seizing up. Use a different nondairy milk such as oat or rice milk, or whole dairy milk, if you like.

4 POPS

⅓ cup (80 g) extra dark chocolate chips

2 Tbsp unsweetened natural cocoa powder

1 cup (250 ml) almond milk

¼ cup (50 g) sugar

2 Tbsp tahini

Four 4-inch (10-cm) wooden ice pop sticks or ice pop molds with handles

In a mixing bowl, combine the chocolate chips and natural cocoa powder.

In a microwaveable container, heat the almond milk to almost boiling. Pour the hot liquid over the chocolate and let sit undisturbed for 1 minute, then whisk until combined. Whisk in the sugar and tahini.

Pour the chocolate mixture into a mold with four 4-fl oz (125-ml) cavities. Freeze the pops until they are firm enough to hold a wooden stick in place. After inserting the sticks, wait until the pops are solid, at least 4 hours, depending on your freezer.

To serve, fill a large bowl with hot water. Hold the mold submerged as far as possible in the water for 2 minutes. The pops should release when tugged slowly and firmly. Running a thin knife around inside the rim of the mold cavities may help. The pops will keep in the mold in the freezer for up to 5 days.

TIP *Tahini, a peanut butter–like paste made from ground sesame seeds, is available near the peanut butter in some supermarkets, at natural food stores, and in Middle Eastern stores. Tahini is made using raw sesame seeds, with a mild nutty taste, or with roasted seeds that taste more intense. Stir it thoroughly before using.*

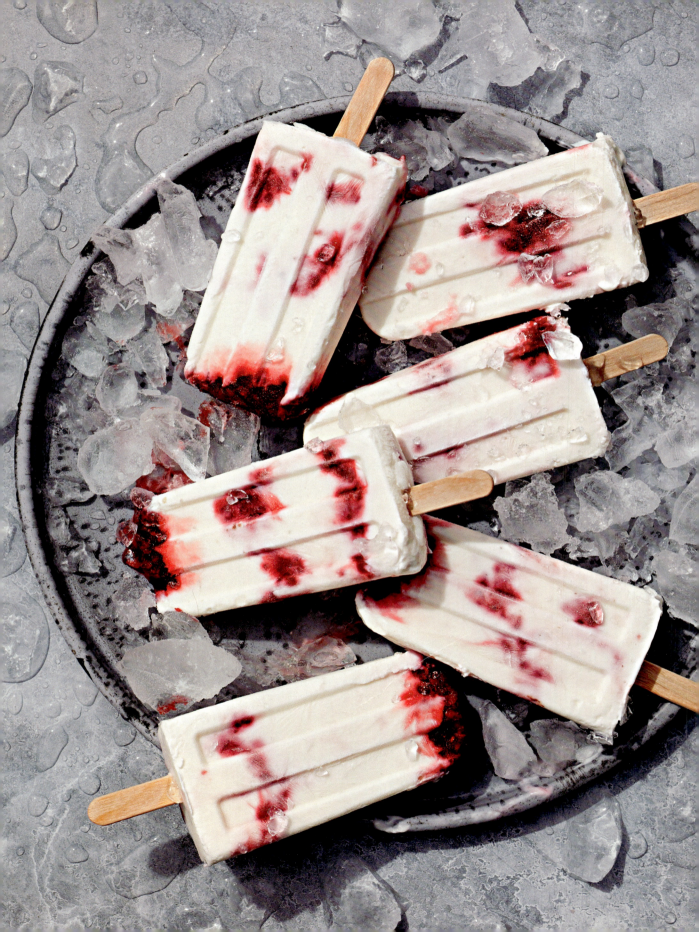

Raspberry Swirl Frozen Yogurt Pops

Greek yogurt makes these creamy pops rich in protein and calcium. It stays nicely creamy when frozen. A touch of honey softens the yogurt's tartness. Even if your raspberries do not swirl perfectly, these energy-boosting pops will still taste grand. In the freezer, you can keep the pops for up to three days.

4 SERVINGS

½ cup (70 g) frozen unsweetened raspberries, partially thawed

2 Tbsp confectioners' sugar

1 ½ cups (375 g) plain whole-milk Greek yogurt

3 Tbsp honey

½ tsp pure vanilla extract

Four 4-inch (10-cm) wooden ice pop sticks or ice pop molds with handles

In a small bowl, mash the partially thawed raspberries with the confectioners' sugar.

In another bowl, combine the yogurt, honey, and vanilla and stir until the mixture is smooth.

Using an ice pop mold with four 4–fl oz (125-ml) cavities, spoon 2 generous tablespoonfuls of the yogurt mixture into the bottom of each cavity. Add 2 tsp of the raspberry mixture. Do this layering twice more.

To create raspberry swirls and streaks, work a thin-bladed knife up and down and twist it in the yogurt. Top off each cavity with the remaining yogurt. Insert a wooden stick into each pop, leaving about 1 inch (2.5 cm) sticking up.

Freeze the pops until solid, about 4 hours.

To unmold, fill a large bowl with hot tap water. Hold the mold in the water for 1 minute. Run the blade of a small knife around the inside between the mold and the yogurt. Using a gentle rocking motion, slowly and firmly pull to release the pops from the mold. Repeat dipping the mold in the hot water, if necessary. Serve right away.

Double Rich Hot Chocolate

Dark, intense, and containing enough caffeine to be a morning eye-opener, this is cocoa for grown-ups. Roasted natural cocoa powder keeps the micronutrients that are lost when the cocoa is Dutch-processed. Using a raw cocoa powder increases this benefit even more. Coconut sugar adds minerals and a caramel note, while vanilla and cinnamon mellow the unsweetened cocoa powder's astringent taste.

2 SERVINGS

1 cup (250 ml) canned unsweetened coconut milk

¼ cup (20 g) unsweetened natural cocoa powder

1 oz (30 g) best quality dark chocolate (70–73 percent cacao), finely chopped

2–3 Tbsp coconut sugar

¼ tsp pure vanilla extract

Ground cinnamon, for garnish

In a measuring cup, combine the coconut milk with 1 cup (250 ml) water.

In a heavy saucepan over medium-low heat, heat ½ cup (125 ml) of the diluted coconut milk until bubbles appear around the edge. Off the heat, whisk in the cocoa powder, chopped chocolate, and sugar to make a creamy ganache. Whisk in the remaining liquid.

Return the pot to the heat and whisk until the liquid is hot, about 4 minutes. Stir in the vanilla.

Divide the hot chocolate between two large mugs. Garnish each serving with a dash of ground cinnamon. Serve right away.

TIP *Look for a coconut milk without added thickeners for the smoothest result.*

Super-Charged Kale Smoothie

All the ingredients in this vibrant green drink are superfoods. They contain a nutrient-dense combination of carbs, healthy fat, protein, and a host of antioxidants, including from the matcha tea. Matcha also contains energizing caffeine, making this smoothie a good morning starter or mid-afternoon reviver. To skip the caffeine, use decaffeinated green tea.

2 SERVINGS

2 cups (500 ml) cold matcha green tea

4 lacinato kale leaves, stemmed, torn into pieces

1 cup (160 g) frozen mango chunks

½ ripe small avocado, cut into chunks

2 Tbsp smooth almond butter

4 pitted dates, coarsely chopped

1 Tbsp chia seeds

1 Tbsp hemp seeds

½-inch (12-mm) piece fresh ginger, peeled and roughly chopped

In a high-powered blender or regular blender, combine the tea, kale, mango, avocado, almond butter, dates, chia and hemp seeds, and ginger. Process until the mixture is smooth, 30–45 seconds. Divide between 2 large glasses, and serve right away.

Watermelon Chia Water

Tiny chia seeds are packed with protein, fiber, and minerals. When they are combined with water, they amp up its revitalizing power. Pairing chia water with watermelon puts it over the top as a workout partner. To avoid diluting its flavor with ice, serve this naturally sweet drink in a chilled glass or sip it from a refillable bottle you have stored in the fridge.

2 SERVINGS

2 Tbsp chia seeds

3 cups (450 g) chilled ripe seedless watermelon cubes

1 Tbsp fresh lime juice

2 sprigs fresh mint

In a jar with a tight-fitting lid, combine 2 cups (500 ml) cold water and the chia seeds. Cover tightly and shake vigorously. Place the jar in the refrigerator for about 20 minutes, shaking it briskly four or five times to keep the chia suspended evenly in the water.

Meanwhile, in a large glass measuring pitcher, use an immersion blender to process the watermelon until liquefied, making 2 cups (500 ml) watermelon juice. (Alternatively, purée the watermelon in a blender.) Add the chilled chia water and lime juice and mix to combine.

Divide between tall chilled glasses, garnish with the mint sprigs, and serve right away.

Golden Turmeric Latte

Almonds and oats both contain tryptophan, an essential amino acid the body uses to regulate sleep and help produce soothing serotonin. This warm drink also contains turmeric and ginger, both rich in antioxidants. Coconut cream adds cozy comfort, making this a perfect nightcap.

2 SERVINGS

2 cups (500 ml) unsweetened oat milk

2 tsp ground turmeric

½ tsp ground cinnamon

⅛ tsp freshly ground black pepper

¼ cup (60 ml) unsweetened coconut cream

2 Tbsp smooth raw almond butter

2 tsp peeled and grated fresh ginger

1 Tbsp honey

2 cinnamon sticks, for garnish (optional)

In a small saucepan over medium heat, warm ¼ cup (60 ml) of the oat milk until bubbles start forming around the edge. Add the turmeric, cinnamon, and black pepper and whisk to make a paste. Pour in the remaining oat milk, the coconut cream, almond butter, ginger, and honey. Heat, whisking until the almond butter dissolves and the latte is hot; do not let it boil.

Divide the hot latte between two large mugs. If desired, with a hand-held milk foamer, froth the top of each latte. Add a cinnamon stick to each mug, if using. Serve right away.

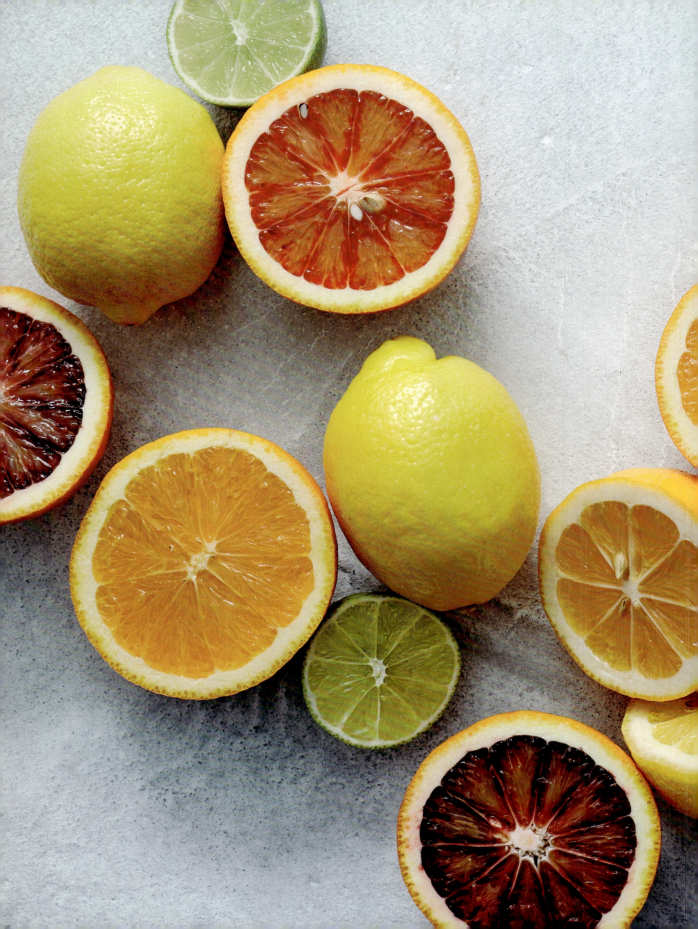

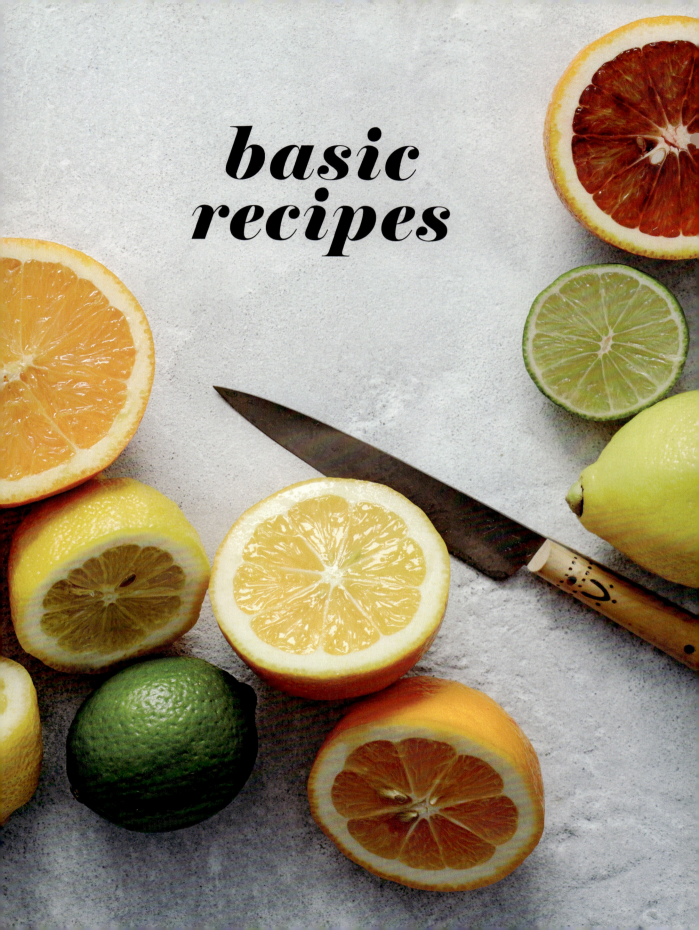

basic recipes

Basic Cooked Rice

4–6 SERVINGS

1 cup (200 g) long-grain white rice

Place the rice in a fine-mesh sieve and rinse under cold running water until the water runs clear. Transfer the rice to a heavy saucepan and add 1 ½ cups (350 ml) water. Cover the pan, place it over high heat, and bring to a boil. Reduce the heat to low and simmer, undisturbed, for about 20 minutes. Remove from the heat and let stand, covered, for 5 minutes. Fluff the rice with a fork and serve right away.

Sesame Brown Rice

4 SERVINGS

1 cup (190 g) medium-grain brown rice
Sea salt
2 tsp sesame seeds
1 tsp toasted sesame oil
1 Tbsp thinly sliced green onion tops

In a saucepan, bring 2 ¾ cups (650 ml) water to a boil over high heat. Add the rice and ½ tsp salt, stir once, and reduce the heat to low. Cover and simmer very gently, without stirring, until all the water has been absorbed and the grains are tender, 35–45 minutes.

Meanwhile, in a small, dry frying pan over medium heat, toast the sesame seeds, stirring constantly, until they are fragrant and have darkened slightly, about 2 minutes. Immediately pour the seeds onto a plate to cool. Set aside.

Carefully lift the cover of the saucepan so that no condensation drips into the rice. Drizzle the sesame oil evenly over the top and sprinkle with half of the sesame seeds. Gently fluff the rice with a fork or the handle of a wooden spoon.

Spoon the rice into a serving dish. Sprinkle with the remaining sesame seeds and the green onion. Serve right away.

Brown Aromatic Rice

4–6 SERVINGS

Brown basmati or jasmine rice, 1⅓ cups (250 g)

In a saucepan, bring 2 cups (500 ml) salted water to a boil over high heat. Add the rice and return to a boil. Reduce the heat to low, cover, and cook for 30 minutes.

Keeping the pan covered, turn off the heat and let stand 5 minutes. Fluff the rice with a fork and serve right away.

Saffron Rice

4–6 SERVINGS

1 Tbsp olive oil
1 small shallot, chopped
1 cup (200 g) basmati rice
Kosher salt
¼ tsp saffron threads, crumbled

In a saucepan over medium-high heat, heat the olive oil. Add the shallot and sauté until translucent, about 2 minutes. Add the rice, 2 cups (500 ml) water, ½ tsp salt, and the saffron and bring to a boil. Reduce the heat to low, cover, and simmer for about 20 minutes. Fluff the rice with a fork and serve right away.

Basic Cooked Quinoa

4–6 SERVINGS

1 cup (180 g) quinoa
Kosher salt and freshly ground black pepper
2 tsp extra-virgin olive oil

Place the quinoa in a sieve and rinse well under cold running water.

In a saucepan, bring 2 cups (500 ml) water to a boil over high heat. Add the rinsed quinoa and ½ tsp salt. Reduce the heat to low, cover, and simmer until the water is absorbed and the quinoa is tender, about 20 minutes.

Drizzle the cooked quinoa with olive oil, season to taste with salt and pepper, and toss well with a fork. Serve right away.

Basic Cooked Bulgur

4–6 SERVINGS

1 cup (150 g) bulgur wheat, quick cooking
Kosher salt

In a saucepan, combine the bulgur and 1 ½ cups (350 ml) cold water. Sprinkle lightly with salt. Bring the water to a boil over high heat. Reduce the heat to low, cover, and simmer until the bulgur is just tender, 12–15 minutes. Turn off the heat and let the bulgur stand, covered, for at least 5 minutes. Fluff the bulgur with a fork and serve right away.

Bulgur & Lentil Pilaf with Almonds

4 SERVINGS

¾ cup (150 g) brown lentils
2 Tbsp olive oil
1 yellow onion, chopped
2 cloves garlic, minced
1 cup (150 g) medium-grain bulgur wheat
1 tsp ground coriander
Kosher salt and freshly ground black pepper
2 cups (500 ml) low-sodium vegetable broth or water
¼ cup (30 g) roasted almonds
⅓ cup (13 g) fresh flat-leaf parsley leaves
1 Tbsp grated lemon zest
2 Tbsp fresh lemon juice

Pick over the lentils for stones or broken or misshapen lentils. Rinse thoroughly under cold running water and drain. In a small saucepan, combine the lentils with water to cover by 2 inches (5 cm) and bring to a boil over medium-high heat. Reduce the heat to medium-low, cover, and simmer gently until tender but firm to the bite, about 20 minutes. Drain thoroughly and set aside.

In a large frying pan over medium-high heat, heat the olive oil. Add the onion and cook, stirring often, until the onion is wilted, 2–3 minutes. Add the garlic, bulgur, coriander, ¼ tsp salt, and ¼ tsp pepper and cook, stirring often, until the garlic is fragrant, about 1 minute. Stir in the lentils and the broth and bring to a boil. Reduce the heat to low, cover, and simmer for 5 minutes. Remove from the heat and let stand, covered, for 15 minutes.

Place the almonds, parsley, and lemon zest on a cutting board and coarsely chop them together. Fluff the pilaf with a fork and stir in the lemon juice. Season to taste with salt and pepper. Mound the pilaf on a serving platter, sprinkle with the almond mixture, and serve right away.

Olive Oil Mashed Potatoes

4–6 SERVINGS

2 lb (1 kg) Yukon Gold potatoes, peeled
Kosher salt and freshly ground black pepper
1 cup (250 ml) milk
3 Tbsp extra-virgin olive oil

Put the potatoes in a large saucepan and add water to cover by 1 inch (2.5 cm). Add 1 tsp salt, place over high heat, and bring the water to a boil. Reduce the heat to low and simmer until the potatoes are tender when pierced with a knife, 25–30 minutes.

In a small saucepan, warm the milk over medium heat just until small bubbles form around the edges of the pan. Remove from the heat and stir in the olive oil.

Drain the potatoes and return to the pot. Using a potato masher, mash the potatoes until smooth. Using a wooden spoon, gently mix in the milk-oil mixture. Season to taste with salt and pepper and serve.

Black Bean Mash

4–6 SERVINGS

1 cup (300 g) dried pinto beans, picked over, rinsed, and soaked in water to cover for at least 4 hours and up to overnight
½ white onion
1 clove garlic
1 bay leaf
2 Tbsp olive oil
Kosher salt

In a large saucepan over high heat, combine the beans, onion, garlic, bay leaf, and water to cover by 2 inches (5 cm) and bring to a boil. Reduce the heat to maintain a low simmer and cook until the beans are very tender, 1–2 hours, depending on the freshness of the beans. Drain the beans, reserving the cooking water, and discard the onion, garlic, and bay leaf.

In a large frying pan over medium heat, heat the olive oil. Add the beans and cook, smashing them with the back of a wooden spoon, until reduced to a lumpy mashed potato–like texture, adding about 1 cup of the reserved cooking water to achieve the desired texture. Season to taste with salt amd keep warm until ready to serve.

Stove-Top Herbed Polenta

4–6 SERVINGS

1 Tbsp olive oil
½ small yellow onion, chopped
Kosher salt and freshly ground black pepper
1 cup (160 g) polenta
¾ cup (3 oz/90 g) coarsely grated Parmesan or pecorino romano cheese
1 Tbsp chopped fresh marjoram or thyme

In a heavy saucepan over medium heat, heat the olive oil. Add the onion and sauté until tender, about 5 minutes. Add 4 cups (1 l) water, 1 tsp salt, and 1 tsp pepper and bring to a boil over high heat.

Gradually whisk in the polenta. Bring the mixture back to a boil, stirring frequently. Reduce the heat to low and simmer slowly, stirring frequently, until the polenta is thick, about 18 minutes. Mix in the cheese and marjoram and serve right away.

Pizza Dough

1½ LB (680 G) DOUGH,
OR ENOUGH FOR 2 PIZZAS

1 cup (250 ml) warm water (105°–100°F/40°–43°C)
1½ tsp active dry yeast
2¾ cups (440 g) unbleached all-purpose flour,
plus more for dusting
3 tbsp vital wheat gluten (pure gluten flour) or bread flour
1½ tsp kosher salt
2 tbsp extra-virgin olive oil, plus more for brushing

In a large glass measuring pitcher, whisk together
the water and yeast. Let stand for 5 minutes.

In a food processor, combine the flour, the wheat
gluten, and the salt and process to mix. Whisk the olive
oil into the yeast mixture. With the processor running,
add the yeast mixture and process until the dough
comes together and forms a ball, about 1 minute.
(If the dough does not form a ball, add water by the
tablespoonful until it comes together.)

Turn out the dough onto a lightly floured work surface
and knead briefly until smooth. Brush a large bowl with
olive oil. Shape the dough into a ball, place it in the
bowl, and turn the dough to coat it with oil. Cover the
bowl with a kitchen towel and let stand until doubled
in volume, about 1 ½ hours.

Punch down the dough and divide in half. Use at once,
or shape each half into a ball, place each ball in a
resealable plastic bag, and refrigerate for up to
2 days or freeze for up to 1 month.

Let the refrigerated dough stand for 1 hour and the
frozen dough thaw for 4 hours at room temperature
before using.

Hummus

ABOUT 3 CUPS (750 G)

2 cups (12 oz/375 g) drained cooked or canned chickpeas
⅓ cup (80 ml) fresh lemon juice, or as needed
¼ cup (75 g) tahini paste
¼ cup (60 ml) plus 1 Tbsp extra-virgin olive oil
2 cloves garlic, finely chopped
Sea salt and freshly ground black pepper
1 Tbsp chopped fresh flat-leaf parsley leaves
1 Tbsp pine nuts
1 tsp ground sumac or paprika

In a food processor or blender, combine the chickpeas,
lemon juice, tahini, ¼ cup (60 ml) of the olive oil, the
garlic, a big pinch of salt, and several grindings of
pepper and process until smooth. If too thick, add

a spoonful of water or lemon juice to achieve the
desired consistency. Taste and adjust the seasoning.
To serve, mound in a bowl and drizzle with the
remaining 1 Tbsp olive oil and sprinkle with the
parsley, pine nuts, and sumac.

Kale Pesto

1 CUP (250 ML)

4 oz (120 g) stemmed and chopped curly kale
(4 packed cups)
3 cloves garlic, chopped (1 Tbsp)
¼ cup (30 g) chopped walnuts
⅓ cup (75 ml) extra-virgin olive oil
3 Tbsp grated Parmesan cheese
Freshly ground black pepper

Place the kale, garlic, and walnuts in a food processor
and pulse until the kale is finely chopped, about
20 pulses. Add the nuts. With the motor running, slowly
drizzle in the olive oil, and continue whirling until the
pesto looks creamy but still has texture. Add the
cheese and pulse to blend. Season with pepper.

Avocado Green Goddess Dressing

ABOUT 1½ CUPS (350 ML)

1 clove garlic
1 small avocado, halved and pitted
2 anchovy fillets in olive oil, minced
½ cup (15 g) packed fresh basil leaves
¼ cup (15 g) coarsely chopped fresh chives
2 Tbsp fresh tarragon
½ tsp Dijon mustard
¾ cup (180 ml) buttermilk
2 Tbsp fresh lemon juice
2 Tbsp extra-virgin olive oil
1–4 Tbsp (15–60 ml) warm water
Kosher salt and freshly ground black pepper

In a food processor with the motor running, drop the
garlic through the feed tube. Turn the processor off and
add the scooped-out avocado flesh, anchovies, basil,
chives, tarragon, and mustard; pulse to combine and
chop the basil finely. With the processor running, slowly
stream in the buttermilk, lemon juice, olive oil, and up
to 4 Tbsp (60 ml) warm water to achieve a pourable
consistency. Season to taste with salt and pepper. Use
immediately, or transfer to an airtight container and
refrigerate for up to 1 week.

Mango-Avocado Salsa

ABOUT 2¼ CUPS (530 ML)

1 ripe mango, diced

1 ripe avocado, halved, pitted, and diced

1 green onion, white and light green parts, thinly sliced

½–1 jalapeño chile, finely minced

2 Tbsp rice vinegar

1 Tbsp extra-virgin olive oil

½ Tbsp hot sauce

Sea salt and freshly ground black pepper

In a bowl, gently mix together all of the ingredients. Season to taste with salt and pepper.

Four-Seed Topping

ABOUT ⅓ CUP (30 G)

2 Tbsp toasted sliced almonds

1 Tbsp raw pumpkin seeds

1 Tbsp sunflower seeds

1 Tbsp toasted sesame seeds

2 tsp chia seeds

On a cutting board, combine the almonds, pumpkin seeds, and sunflower seeds and chop coarsely. Place the chopped nuts and seeds in a small bowl. Add the sesame seeds and chia seeds. The topping will keep for up to 1 week, tightly covered in the refrigerator.

Warm Berry Compote

4 SERVINGS

¼ cup (60 g) sugar

2 cups (250 g) strawberries, hulled and quartered

1 cup (125 g) blueberries

1 cup (125 g) blackberries

1 tsp fresh lemon juice

Pinch of sea salt

2 tablespoons unsalted butter, at room temperature, cut into cubes

In a large, nonreactive sauté pan over medium heat, combine the sugar and ¼ cup (60 ml) water and bring to a boil, stirring to dissolve the sugar.

Cook for 2 minutes, then add the strawberries, blueberries, blackberries, lemon juice, and salt. Return to a boil, add the butter, and swirl the mixture in the pan until the butter melts. Serve right away.

Lemon Kissed Strawberry Jam

ABOUT 1 HALF-PINT JAR (250-ML)

1 lb (500 g) strawberries, hulled

½ cup (100 g) sugar

½ tsp grated lemon zest

1 tsp fresh lemon juice

Put the berries in a heavy saucepan. Using a potato masher, roughly mash them, leaving some berries whole. Place over medium heat and simmer, stirring occasionally, until reduced to about 1 cup (250 ml), about 12 minutes.

Meanwhile, in a small bowl, rub the sugar and lemon zest together between your fingertips to release the essential oils in the zest. When the strawberries are ready, add the lemon sugar and continue cooking, stirring frequently, until the mixture thickens and is reduced again to 1 cup (250 ml), about 6 minutes. Stir in the lemon juice.

Transfer the jam to a clean jar, cap tightly, and refrigerate for up to 2 weeks.

Roasted Pear Butter

ABOUT 1½ CUPS (350 ML)

2 Tbsp unsalted butter, melted, plus more for greasing

5 small Bosc or Comice pears (about 1 ½ lb/680 g total weight)

2 Tbsp firmly packed light brown sugar

2 Tbsp honey

Position a rack in the lower third of the oven and preheat to 400°F (200°C). Grease a large rimmed baking sheet with butter.

Peel, quarter, and core the pears, then cut each quarter in half crosswise. In a bowl, combine the pears and the 2 Tbsp melted butter and toss to coat evenly. Spread the pears in a single layer on the prepared baking sheet. Sprinkle the brown sugar evenly over the pears.

Roast the pears until tender when pierced with a small, sharp knife and browned on the edges, about 30 minutes. Remove from the oven and transfer the pears and all the caramelized juices on the bottom of the pan to a food processor. Let stand until cool.

Process the cooled pears until smooth. Add the honey and process to combine. Transfer the pear butter to a clean jar, cap tightly, and refrigerate for up to 2 weeks.

the healthy ingredient glossary

The Good Food for Good Health section on pages 8–15 lays out major food groups and the different healthy benefits they provide. Here, you will find details on many of the healthy ingredients mentioned there or used in the recipes throughout this book.

ALMONDS contain the highest amount of monounsaturated fat, the kind also found in olive oil, and the most fiber of all nuts. One ounce (28 g) provides as much protein as an egg. Their tan skin contains most of the almond's antioxidants. Use almonds as a nutrition-boosting topping on salads, vegetables, and muffins. Almond flour helps make Double Almond Waffles with Fresh Berry Salsa (page 150) gluten-free.

AVOCADO OIL is pressed from avocado pulp. It consists mainly of oleic acid, a heart-healthy omega-9 fatty acid. Avocado oil is growing in popularity thanks to studies showing it lowers blood cholesterol. It's also rich in lutein, an antioxidant that protects vision. Avocado oil is stable at high heat, making it a great choice for sautéing and stir-frying.

BARLEY is high in fiber that helps lower cholesterol. Cook it like risotto, like porridge, or like rice. Or, make classic Mushroom Barley Soup with Fresh Thyme (page 40).

BASIL LEAVES are delicate, but this member of the mint family is rich in anti-inflammatory and anti-bacterial benefits from phytonutrients, including limonene and eugenol. Basil is rich in vitamins A, C, and K, which helps blood to clot and bones to stay strong. Use fresh basil rather than dried to best enjoy this aromatic herb's anise, mint, and citrus notes.

BEEF is rich in B vitamins and minerals, including zinc and selenium, and when eaten in moderation can be part of a healthy diet. It is a source of B-12, an essential vitamin found only in animal foods that is vital for good energy, a healthy nervous system, and the ability to make red blood cells. Compared to conventionally raised meat, grass-fed beef is leaner and has more omega-3 fatty acids as well as conjugated linoleic acid (CLA), another useful anti-inflammatory.

BULGUR, which is whole grain wheat that is steamed, dried, and cracked, stars in tabbouleh. Coarse bulgur is particularly fiber-rich and a good source of B vitamins. Its nutty taste enhances Bulgur & Lentil Pilaf with Almonds (page 185).

CAYENNE PEPPER gets its heat from capsaicin, a compound that speeds up metabolism, helps clear the lungs when you have a cold, and even fights cancer. Cayenne's bright red color comes from antioxidants lycopene and astaxanthin. It is rich with vitamins A, C, and E, riboflavin, folate, magnesium, and potassium. Using a pinch brightens flavor without adding heat, a nice and healthy touch in all kinds of dishes.

CHEESE can be a smart addition to a meal, contributing protein, calcium, and beneficial bacteria (since cheese is fermented). Low-moisture cheeses are higher in protein and lower in fat than other kinds. Italian Parmigino-Reggiano, made using partially skimmed milk from grass-fed cows, is more digestible than other cheeses. It adds rich umami flavor to pasta and vegetable dishes, or shaved over a green salad, and its rind is edible; simmer a piece in soup to enrich its flavor. Aged pecorino, made from sheep's milk, comes mainly from Rome, Sardinia, or Sicily. Its sharp, salty flavor means a little adds a lot of flavor, especially to pasta dishes. Feta, most often made from shweep's milk, adds tangy flavor when crumbled over salads or pasta. People who have problems digesting cow's milk cheese may find cheeses made with these other milks easier on the system.

CHIA SEEDS contain fiber that may help lower the risk of type 2 diabetes by stabilizing blood sugar levels. Their omega-3s help reduce the inflammation associated with heart disease. Whirl chia seeds in smoothies, mix them into Watermelon Chia Water (page 180), and combine with your favorite nut milk to make a creamy pudding.

CHICKEN is considered a lean meat and thus a good low-fat protein source; it provides all nine essential amino acids and also contains phosphorous and calcium. Cage-free chickens wander only indoors. Free-range and organic birds get outdoor access, often through a small opening at one end of the barn, and limited outside space. Pastured birds spend days outside roaming and scratching. Pastured chicken has more vitamins A, E, and omega-3s. Air-chilled chicken has better flavor and texture than conventionally processed birds.

CHILE FLAKES are made by crushing dried small red chile peppers. These peppers contain less capsaicin, making them milder than cayenne. Include the seeds along with the flakes for maximum heat. Chili flakes sprinkled liberally on dishes stimulate your brain enough to release mood-lifting endorphins.

CILANTRO has remarkable properties, including the ability to kill salmonella bacteria, thanks to a natural antimicrobial compound, dodecenal. It also is rich in vitamins A, C, and K; potassium; calcium; and the antioxidant micronutrient quercetin. Cilantro is widely used in Asian, Middle Eastern, and South American cooking. Tossing a handful of cilantro leaves into a green salad adds an interesting note. Heat diminishes cilantro's flavor, so add it later in cooked dishes or use it as a garnish.

CINNAMON coming from Vietnam and Indonesia tastes more intense, pungent, and less sweet than cinnamon from Ceylon. It looks redder, too. It is actually cassia, a different plant. Ceylon cinnamon botanically is true cinnamon. It tastes mellow and earthy. Cassia bark makes cinnamon sticks that appear thicker and rougher than the smooth surface of true cinnamon bark sticks. Both true cinnamon

and cassia help lower blood sugar levels and contain an aromatic trio of antibacterial oils. Ceylon cinnamon is ideal in savory dishes while cassia goes well in baking and desserts.

COCONUT OIL adds rich flavor, especially in Asian cooking. It's high in a type of saturated fat, known as medium-chain triglycerides, that boosts fat burning and may help raise good HDL cholesterol. Lauric acid in coconut oil can kill bacteria, and coconut oil makes an excellent skin moisturizer! Refined coconut oil is best for high-heat cooking.

COD is a good source of omega-3s; vitamin B-6, important for metabolic processes; and vitamin B-12, which supports nerve and blood cells. It is also versatile, good in curries and soups, or simply baked with lemon and olive oil.

CUMIN contains antioxidants that help boost your immune system and improve cognition. It also aids digestion. Cumin contains a wide range of vitamins (A, C, E, and several B vitamins), manganese needed for several body functions, potassium, zinc, and more. It is the love-or-hate spice, much as cilantro is the love-or-hate herb: your reaction to its dry, earthy flavor with citrus and pepper notes is genetic. Cooks in North African, Latin America, and Asia, especially India, use both ground cumin and the whole seed.

EDAMAME, the bright green soybeans sold frozen in the pod or shelled, are loaded with fiber and protein. Boil the pods in salted

water for a great snack or to munch as protein-to-go. Use shelled edamame in salads, stir-fries, and side dishes.

FARRO is an ancient, unhybridized form of wheat. Cook it like rice to serve warm as pilaf or at room temperature in salads. Farro ground into flour is used to make whole-grain pasta.

FLAX SEEDS are rich in essential fatty acids that help lower the risk of stroke and promote heart health by reducing bad blood cholesterol. They are uniquely rich in lignans, phytonutrients that help lower risk of breast, prostate, and other cancers. These and other benefits are most available in ground flax meal. In vegan baking, 2 tablespoons ground flax can replace an egg.

GINGER has a very long list of proven health benefits, including reducing nausea and inhibiting the body's production of inflammatory substances that cause arthritis pain. Its heat comes from gingerol, a compound related to capsaicin. It also is rich in vitamin C, magnesium, potassium, and copper. Use the edge of a spoon to peel fresh ginger. Then grate it on a rasp or add whole slices to soups, stews, and stir-frys. Dried ground ginger plays an important role in baking but is not a great substitute for fresh, as they taste quite different.

GRAPESEED OIL is a polyunsaturated oil high in omega-6 fatty acids. Its high smoke point is good for stir-frying and sautéing. Chefs like its neutral taste for baking and salad dressings.

continued following page

HEMP SEEDS are rich in protein, antioxidant vitamin E, and polyunsaturated fat. They contain argenine, an amino acid that produces nitric acid in the body that helps keep blood vessels open and flexible. Add them to smoothies, sprinkle on salads, and blend them into hummus.

KIMCHI is a pungent Korean pickled cabbage that gets its strong flavors from hot chiles and lots of garlic, plus ginger, salt, and fish sauce. Made with napa cabbage, it may include daikon radish, cucumber, or a combination. Vegan kimchi skips the fish sauce. Along with live probiotics that aid digestion, kimchi is rich in fiber, capsaicin from the chile pepper, and antioxidants in garlic and ginger.

LAMB is a rich source of protein, as well as vitamin B-12, iron, and zinc, which are immune system boosters. It does contain a high quantity of saturated fat (more than pork), so is not the best heart-healthy choice. Lamb grazes so it is mostly grass-fed and lean; it can be organic.

MILK is a good source of absorbable calcium for many people. (Calcium in milk is more absorbable than that from beans, spinach, and sweet potatoes, but less absorbable than that from broccoli, kale, and bok choy.) A glass contains more protein than one egg, and it provides vitamin A, riboflavin, and vitamin B-12. Most milk is fortified with vitamin D, which, together with calcium, is important for strong bones. Comparing reduced-fat (2%), low fat (1%), and whole milk, reduced fat has more protein and about one-third less saturated fat than

whole. Whole milk contains less carbohydrate, in the form of milk sugars, and more omega-3s than lower-fat milks, and it can contribute a feeling of satiety that prevents snacking. In other words, each has its advantages, so choose the milk that works for you! Organic milk contains more omega-3s and provides a better ratio of omega-3 to omega-6 fat than regular milk, along with higher concentrations of vitamin E, selenium, and carotenoids.

MINT contains menthol, a natural decongestant, and rosmarinic acid, an anti-inflammatory helpful during allergy season. Mint tea made by steeping fresh mint leaves or a tea bag in hot water is a good way to take advantage these benefits. Essential oils in mint aid digestion, so also sip mint tea after meals. Sharp, bitter peppermint is stimulating, while mild, sweet spearmint feels soothing. Dried crushed mint and fresh mint leaves are often used in Mediterranean cooking.

MISO, famously used to make the Japanese soup, is a bean paste made by fermenting soybeans or other beans, usually together with rice or another grain. Rich in protein and umami flavor, miso is good in salad dressing or barbecue sauce. Try adding a dollop to your tomato sauce! Korean and Chinese cooks use forms of fermented bean paste similar to miso.

MUSSELS are rich in zinc, which helps strengthen your immune system. They rival red meat in iron and folic acid content. As a plus, mussels are sustainably farmed.

OATS are a great source of both soluble fiber, which helps lower blood cholesterol, and insoluble fiber, which promotes good digestion. They are perfect for morning porridge, granola, and for topping a fruit crisp or crumble. For variety, use old-fashioned, thick-cut, or quick-cooking rolled oats, or nubbly steel cut oats: all types are whole grain. Gluten-free oats can be substituted any time in recipes calling for oats.

OLIVE OIL contains the best ratio of antioxidant fatty acids that help raise good cholesterol and lower bad cholesterol. The more peppery olive oil tastes, the more antioxidant polyphenols it contains. Heat destroys these antioxidants, so save your best-flavored extra-virgin olive oil for dressings, drizzling, and quick sautés. However, don't shy away from using regular olive oil for cooking. Resisting unhealthy oxidation at a high heat better than extra-virgin oil, it's a good choice for sautéing and frying.

OREGANO is an essential flavor in Italian cooking and another relative of mint (and a close cousin of marjoram). It contains eugenol and thymol, antibacterials strong enough to kill staph. It is rich in vitamins E and K, B-6, and iron, plus calcium and magnesium needed for good bones. Fresh oregano is sturdy enough to add early in cooking, like dried.

PAPRIKA is made from sweet red bell peppers, hot red peppers, and any other red peppers the producer decides to include. Four different carotenoid antioxidants give it vibrant color. Together with vitamin A, they make paprika beneficial for healthy eyes and skin. Hungarian paprika ranges from sweet to hot. Spanish paprika, also known as pimentón, adds great smoky flavor and depth to vegetarian dishes. It can be found in sweet or hot versions, too.

PARSLEY contains as much iron as spinach and three times the vitamin C in oranges. It is loaded with carotenoids, phytonutrients important for eye health, and copper, needed for normal metabolic processes. It also contains a rich cocktail of antioxidants and volatile oils. The flat-leaf kind tastes better and contains more phytonutrients than curly parsley.

POLENTA must be made from stone-ground corn to be considered whole grain. Yellow polenta contains carotenoids that protect your eyes and heart. Corn is also a good source of thiamin, good for the nervous system, and niacin, which helps regulate blood cholesterol.

PORK contains more fat than beef but has greater amounts of healthy fats. Pork loin and tenderloin are lean, good choices. Small producers are likely to raise pigs most humanely, with less environmental pollution. Pork can be organic.

PUMPKIN SEEDS deliver eight grams of protein in an ounce. Rich in polyunsaturated omega-3 fat, they are also an excellent source of magnesium that helps regulate blood pressure and aids sleep. Include them in granola, on oatmeal, over salads, and sprinkle them over vegetable side dishes.

QUINOA is botanically a seed that we eat like a grain. This pleasantly grassy-tasting South American native is versatile, light, and rich in protein. Serve it at breakfast, in salads, and in main and side dishes. It is used to make excellent gluten-free pasta.

SALMON is a top choice for omega-3s. It's often called a superfood, since thanks to its abundance of quality protein, vitamins, and minerals, including B vitamins, potassium, and selenium, it benefits nearly every system in the body.

SESAME SEEDS are a rich source of calcium needed for healthy bones and nerves, and fiber. Whole sesame seeds, with their beige hull, are most nutritious. Toasting sesame seeds brings out their flavor, making them great as a topping on muffins as well as on savory dishes. Toasted sesame oil adds nutty flavor in Asian dishes.

SHRIMP, like salmon, gets its bright color from astaxanthin, a super antioxidant. It is also a good source of selenium, a mineral that may help reduce inflammation and promote heart health.

TAMARI, a Japanese version of soy sauce, is vegan and usually gluten-free. Made from fermented soybeans, tamari adds welcome umami, or savory flavor, to dishes. Tamari contains less salt than regular soy sauce and is available in reduced-sodium versions.

THYME simmering in soup makes your house smell like a Mediterranean villa. Thyme tea mixed with honey helps loosen and soothe a cough, while antiseptic thymol attacks the bugs making you cough. Yet another mint relative, thyme also gets antioxidant benefits from vitamin C, along with B vitamins, potassium, and zinc. When cooking with fresh thyme, instead of plucking the leaves, toss in whole sprigs tied together to make removing them easy.

TOFU comes in varied textures, from soft and creamy to extra firm and grainy. Cubes or slices of firm tofu go with flavorful sauces, from curry to spicy tomato, and are great for grilling. Pan-crisping firm tofu makes it nicely chewy. Soft tofu is good in Tofu Kimchi Stew (page 43). For a vegan meal, tofu can replace animal ingredients, often suggested in recipes here.

TURMERIC, a cousin of ginger, contains curcumin, one of nature's most potent anti-inflammatories. The more intense its golden orange color, the more concentrated turmeric's power. Used in Indian and Chinese medicine for thousands of years, turmeric can be as effective as over-the-counter medications against inflammation that causes swelling and joint pain. But you have to eat a lot of it, together with black pepper to help your body absorb the curcumin. Turmeric's bitter taste melds beautifully into tomato sauce, lentils, and winter squash dishes.

WALNUTS are rich in polyunsaturated fat and the only nut containing omega-3 essential fatty acids. And the only nut containing ellagic acid, a potent cancer-fighting antioxidant. Whirling walnuts with walnut oil makes a creamy nut butter.

YOGURT provides gut-nurturing bacteria that boost your immune system. Always look for yogurt containing live cultures, with less added sugar. If made using the milk of grass-fed cows, yogurt may contain twice the levels of omega-3 fat than when made with conventional milk.

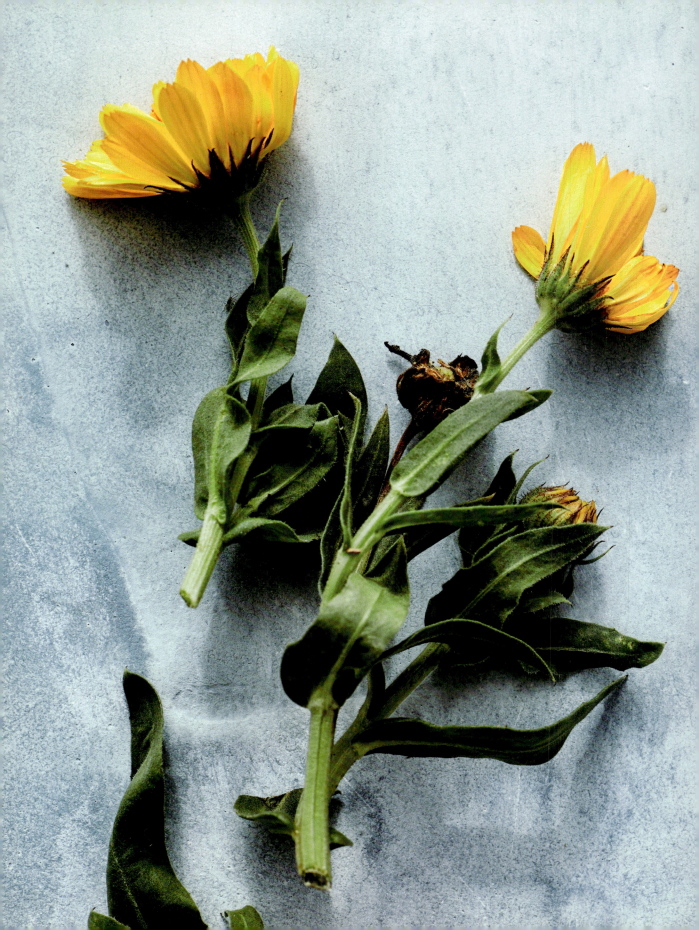

Index

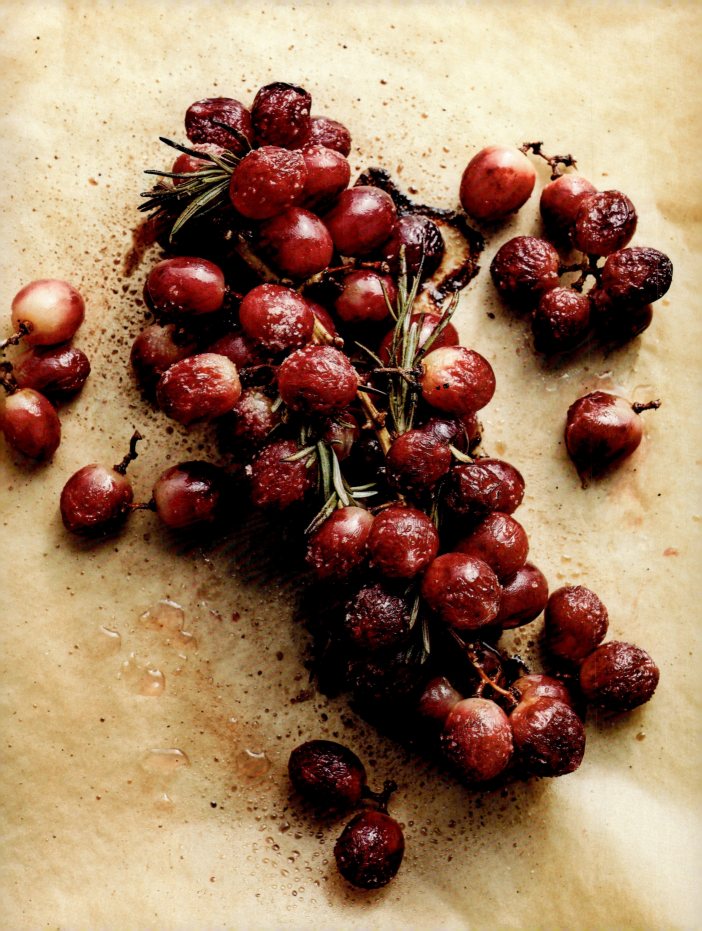

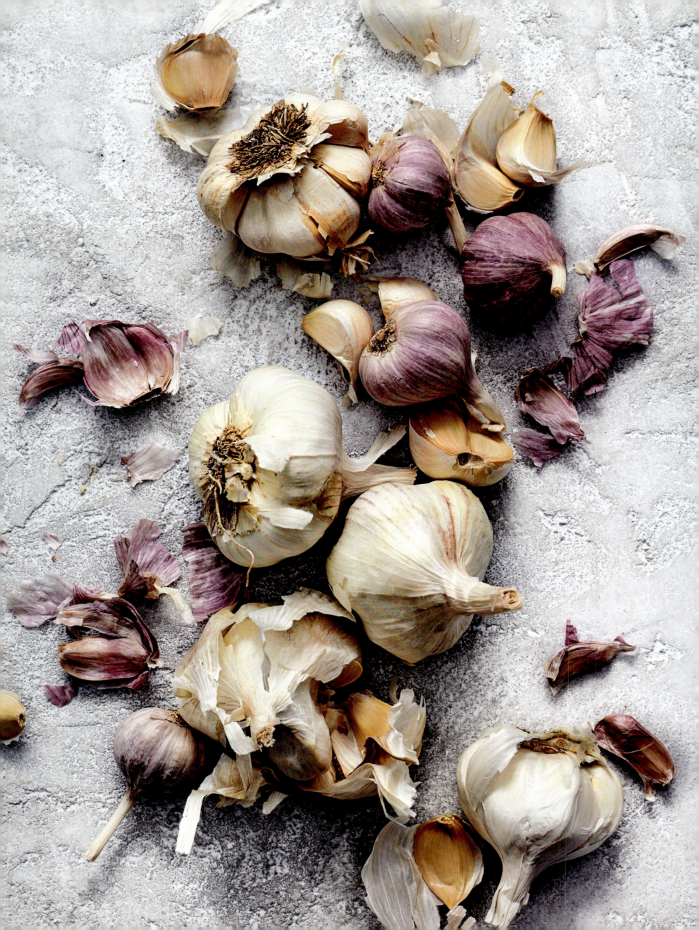

EVERYDAY HEALTHY

weldon**owen**

Produced by Weldon Owen International
1150 Brickyard Cove Road, Richmond, CA 94801
www.weldonowen.com

CEO Raoul Goff
President Kate Jerome
Publisher Roger Shaw
Associate Publisher Amy Marr
Photo Art Director Marisa Kwek
Art Director Bronwyn Lane
Managing Editor Tarji Rodriguez
Production Manager Binh Au
Imaging Manager Don Hill

Photographer Eva Kolenko
Food Stylists Erin Quon
Prop Stylist Claire Mack

Printed and bound in China
First printed in 2020
10 9 8 7 6 5 4 3 2 1

Conceived and produced by
Weldon Owen International
In collaboration with
Williams Sonoma, Inc.
3250 Van Ness Avenue
San Francisco, CA 94109

A WELDON OWEN PRODUCTION

Library of Congress
Cataloging-in-Publication
data is available.

ISBN: 978-1-68188-500-1

ACKNOWLEDGMENTS

Weldon Owen wishes to thank the following people
for their generous support in producing this book:

Sarah Putman Clegg, Alicia Deal, Belle English, Devon Francis,
Josephine Hsu, Eve Lynch, Lori Nunokawa, Elizabeth Parson,
Alisha Petro, Jourdan Platz, Raymond Rudolph, and Alexandra Zeigler.

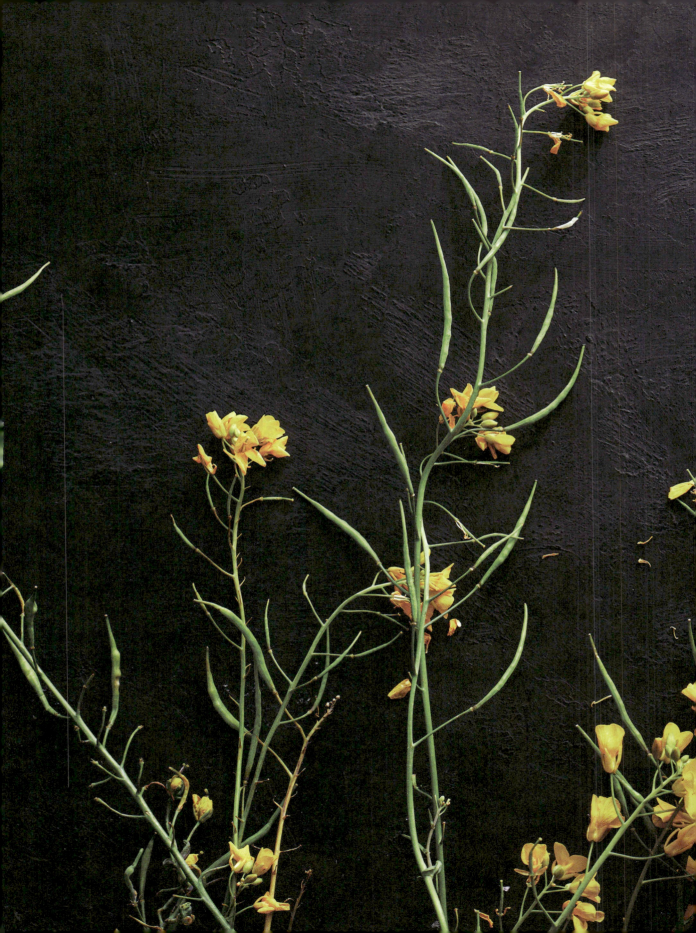